Obesity, Diabetes &
How To Eat To Live

2nd Edition

Transcending the Dietary Dark Ages

Kevin A. Muhammad

TechDoc, Incorporated
Newark, Delaware

Obesity, Diabetes & How To Eat To Live, Transcending the Dietary Dark Ages
2nd Edition

Published in the United States by:
TechDoc, Incorporated
35 Stature Drive
Newark, Delaware 19713
www.etechpublish.com

Printed in the United States of America.

Book design by Kevin A. Muhammad
Cover design by Kevin A. Muhammad, Jr.
Copyedited by Marcia Muhammad

Printed in the United States of America
Main entry under title:
Obesity, Diabetes & How To Eat To Live, Transcending the Dietary Dark Ages, 2nd Edition

A TechDoc book
graphics; tables; charts; pp. 160

Library of Congress Card No. 97-061410
ISBN: 0-9658864-4-1

Appreciation

I bear witness to and appreciate the fact that encompassing and accompanying any good work are numerous realities, both seen and unseen. Although my name, as the author, is on this work, the unseen and most important realities of this work are God, Himself; and those who have shaped and continue to shape my life that I might be used in this way — to be of those who represent the Presence and Work of Almighty God.

As the Giver of all life, all praise, honor, and glory belongs to Almighty (God) Allah. I thank Allah, Who Came In The Person of Master Fard Muhammad, for Giving Humanity Divine Guides in the Persons of the Honorable Elijah Muhammad and the Honorable Minister Louis Farrakhan. I also thank each of these Men for what they have done and continue to do for my family and for me.

I thank my beloved family — wife, Marcia; and children, Kevin, Jr., and Krystina for their great love and support, and for their labor in making this book possible. I also thank my mother, Helen Owens; my twin brother, Julian Muhammad; and my sister, Vernice Mingledoff, for their love, encouragement and generosity.

I also thank Brother Minister Robert Muhammad and the wonderful Believers of Muhammad Mosque No. 35, (Wilmington, Delaware) for their encouragement and support.

Dedication

This book is dedicated to the members of the human family who seek to overcome obesity and chronic disease; and who are in pursuit of optimum health and longevity. This book is a testimony of the Guidance that can help achieve those outcomes — *How To Eat To Live, (Books 1 & 2)*, written by the Honorable Elijah Muhammad.

Other books by Kevin A. Muhammad

Nuts Are Not Good for Humans: Biological Consequences of Consumption

The Slave Diet, Disease & Reparations

Whose Protein? The Value of the Soybean and Navy Bean to Human Nutrition: A Comparative Study

FAQs about How To Eat To Live, Volume One

FAQs about How To Eat To Live, Volume Two

Visit *www.etechpublish.com* for more information.

Contents

Introduction

This is the second edition of *Obesity, Diabetes & How To Eat To Live*. Because the first edition was not widely distributed, it is prudent to restate the motive behind writing this book.

The impetus for writing the first edition, published in 1997, was two-fold. First, it was to alert the public to the forthcoming assault on those suffering from obesity. During the mid-1990s, debates about the cause of obesity began to surface more readily throughout the mass media. So-called health researchers and experts constantly wrangled about this subject. Just as common were the constant release of epidemiological reports and studies about how fat Americans and others around the world were becoming — that obesity was a global pandemic.

Before then, obesity was taboo to discuss in public forums. Few people wanted to consider the subject, not to think of conversing openly about it. This was part of the problem. People detested the subject so much so that they were reluctant to discuss it, even with family members who were suffering from this condition. They turned the other way, and failed to warn their loved ones about the dangers of obesity. The result of this was that families experienced the perils of obesity. Many obese persons, ultimately, succumbed to heart failure and other chronic diseases.

Concurrently, the mass media dared not take up the subject of obesity for fear of reduced ratings. Some national media groups mentioned it occasionally, but superficially. No real media programming addressed the issue. However, in the 1990s, that changed dramatically. The subject began to appear almost hourly. Something *fishy* was happening.

That "something" was the overriding issue of how to define obesity — is it a disease, genetic disorder, or physiological adaptation? Why the sudden interest in obesity from this premise? For the well-aware person, there was little doubt that the *commercial interests* were laying the groundwork for the influx of toxic potions, pills, brutal surgical procedures, and bogus diet plans into the marketplace, as solutions for this crisis.

With the advent of molecular and genetic engineering underway, obesity was the best vehicle to secure government support for research and drug development funding.[1] Major pharmaceutical and biotech companies began putting obesity drugs in the pipeline. Some drugs were ready for release as soon as public sentiment became more amenable to discussing the subject. Obesity was forecasted as the medical industry's new and reemerging *cash-cow*, having long-term, even perpetual, milking potential. To date, the suspicious rise in both *super obesity* and *childhood obesity* ensure that this cash-cow will be milked for decades to come.

The second motivation for the first edition was to reaffirm to the reader that diet was still the best way to eliminate obesity, in spite of the hoopla being made about the new obesity treatments — pills, potions and surgery. It was apparent that the public lacked two important pieces of information that could aid them in the quest to obtain normal weight and better health.

The first piece was the biological workings of the human body. For example, how many people have an understanding of the digestive, circulatory and respiratory systems that is adequate enough to help them make decisions about their health? Unfortunately, the attitude of many people is that this essential knowledge is only for medical practitioners, and that unless you are in the medical field, you have no need of this knowledge. This disposition is ridiculous given the fact that each of us has a body we are responsible for maintaining.

A thorough knowledge of human anatomy and physiology empowers people. We gain a better understanding of health, and what it means to have or not have good health. This knowledge is more empowering than a health plan. Again, such knowledge enables people to actively participate in their own healthcare decisions. Without this knowledge, they are vulnerable to fall for any trick or ill-treat. They leave the entire assessment and treatment decisions to the doctors. This is unfair to doctors. This is unfair to them, as well.

Divine guidance was the other essential body of information that many, if not most, people lacked. To some extent, this remains the case. The reason for this is more obvious today than it was decades ago. Simply put, this is the work of the *merchants of death*. Through their heinous efforts, people are oblivious to Almighty God's interests in all their affairs — eating habits, food preparation and general behavior.

The *merchants of death*, who also conjure religion, use deception to make sure that God is not viewed as real enough for people to place Him in their kitchen, in their bedrooms, in their schools, and in their marketplaces. God is absent from the lives of many people, in that we make Him part of our daily decisions. We need only consider how many times each of us consult Him before making even the most seemingly insignificant decisions.

When knowing that Almighty God is interested in every aspect of our lives, then we incline to Him. We seek, follow and adopt His ways and plan for our lives. Without this real view, we leave life's most important decisions to our own imaginations or in the hands of those who seek profit at our expense. Both these positions comprise today's climate, which has been and remains destructive to human life.

This second edition, *Obesity, Diabetes & How To Eat To Live: Transcending the Dietary Dark Ages*, positions the obesity pandemic in the context of a global disintegration of civilization. This collapse is into a broad darkness that represents a dark age. Marc Widdowson, in his book, *The Phoenix Principle and the Coming Dark Age*, explains dark age. He writes:

> *A dark age is a melting pot when the old, corrupted and exhausted institutions of a failed society are finally broken down and destroyed. Something new and better suited to human needs can then be built up in their place.*

This is the terrain. By now, there should be little doubt that *old, corrupt* and *exhausted* institutions govern the people. Nearly everything seems to be imploding because of corruption and scandal. The enormous morbidity and mortality rates, coupled with the colossal monetary expenditures doled out to address these rates, serve as proof of this.

These systems are supposed to support life, liberty, and the pursuit of happiness, which is not merely limited to certain rights — for example, the right to curse out a person in public via free speech; the right to vote for a controlled and self-serving politician; or the right to carry a gun to rob and kill others. The quality of the population's health is a certain indicator that happiness and liberty is unfettered by tyranny. The fact that poor health is pandemic means that tyranny is present. Again, this is the terrain.

Not knowing this makes it difficult to maneuver therein. Additionally, people must be guided in how best to evade the deadly traps that pervade society. Billions of people remain unable to successfully navigate through the nasty decline of this society. Consequently, they are entangled in the dark mess.

Solving the obesity crisis, therefore, rests on the public's awareness of a terrain that has greed as its topsoil and knowledge of the truth. This truth includes the best means to acquire and maintain good health.

This book describes the pathologies of obesity and diabetes, and the diabolical social and environmental factors that contribute to them. This critical information is contained in chapters 1 through 5.

More importantly, this book reveals that Divine Guidance, which represents the incoming civilization, where longevity, good health, and disease-free living are easily attainable. This Guidance emphatically empowers us. It enables us to evade the deadly entanglement of the *old*, *corrupted* and *exhausted* institutions of this failed society, while preparing us to participate in the rise of the incoming and Divinely-guided civilization.

Chapter 6 details this Guidance, while Chapter 7 provides lifestyle recommendations that aid in the prevention of obesity and diabetes.

CHAPTER 1

Obesity Crises: Historical Insight

The Honorable Elijah Muhammad taught:

History, of all our studies is most and best qualified to reward our research, as it develops the springs and motives of human actions and displays the consequence of circumstances which operate most powerfully upon the destiny of human beings.

So, examination of history is the first place to begin the research of any subject impacting the lives of human beings. Researching the history of obesity allows us to assess this health condition in yesteryear, and what produced it, and then compare it to the dynamics of today. In this, we can arrive at several conclusions.

First, we can determine if the solutions rendered yesteryear to address the obesity crisis worked or if they are on the road to eventually solving the epidemic. Secondly, we can determine if the citizenry simply abandoned the solutions, thus incurring the blame for this continued plight. Finally, we can adjudge whether the population is party to a diabolical scheme of national or global proportion, making them victims of deception, unbeknown to them.

The prevalence of overweight and obesity are fixtures in American society, and has been since the United States was established in the 1700s. In fact, obesity is more common to American life than apple pie and baseball. Gluttony may be the true national pastime.

Some historians implore that obesity was not recognized as a negative condition until after the turn of the 20th century.[2] Before that time, obesity or overweight was fashionable, particularly as it pertained to women. A portly woman was more desired, as the consensus was that plump or fat women were healthy and strong. Thinness was seen as weak, so thin women were less desired.

Of course, this is quite the opposite, today. This turnaround began in the early 1900s, after French designer, Paul Poiret, introduced a new body-revealing style for women. Fatness was now unwanted and thinness became the norm. So, it was not until men began to uncover women in public, removing women's modest way of dressing, that thinness became the standard body type. Now the extremely skinny-body style is considered the standard. This is all one big game, with women as the plaything.

The obesity epidemic epitomizes that old adage *"if you do not learn the lessons of history, you are doomed to repeat it"*. This means that events or conditions are recycled. So, although the obesity epidemic has attracted much attention over the past several decades, this travesty is not new nor is the alarm that it has become an epidemic new. The thing that makes it appear new is the continuous recycling of obesity-related dietary advice, articles, reports, epidemiological studies, medicines, nostrums and fact-finding commissions — rendered by a continuously new breed of health practitioners, researchers, quacks, and politicians.

This recycling process is primarily possible because the average lifespan of the general population is too short. Few people live long enough to say, "I've seen this same nonsense 100 years ago, and it didn't work." As a result, each generation confronts the same problems, and the contemporaries responsible for solving these problems offer the same failed solutions as those before them. Both arise from a system of thinking that is the same today, as it was 100, 200, or 500 years ago.

In the historical context of obesity, we need only examine a short window of time to confirm the "problem/failed-solution" recycling process. The following from James Harvey Young's book, *Medical Messiahs*, exemplifies this fact, while describing the cause of this historical plight during the 1800s.[3] He writes:

> *City eating habits aggravated the widespread biliousness — renamed dyspepsia...For the dietary dark ages still prevailed and developed a deeper gloom among the urban poor. The belief was widespread that all foods contained one 'universal element' which kept life going, so quantity and not quality was stressed. Over-eating was a national habit, an evil compounded by a diet stressing starchy dishes, salt-cured meats, and fat-fried foods.*

This health travesty opened the floodgates for quackery. Purges became popular and every Tom, Dick and Harry seeking to make a quick buck jumped at the opportunity to put forth bogus remedies.

Mr. Young continues:

> *The unabated suffering from countless ailments, rapid growth in the population of the expanding nation, the spirit of therapeutic laissez-faire in a democratic age, the constant growth of media for advertising, legislation that could be turned to good account — all these were factors broadening the market for vendors of packaged remedies.*

Meanwhile, obesity — once considered a semblance of good health — became the target of disdain. With an obese population now feeling shamed, anything that promised a quick cure sold off the shelves. The cures for dyspepsia became cures for obesity.[4] Bogus remedies, with glorified names, such as *Digestives, Human Ease, Densmore's Corpulency Cure, Scott's Emulsion, Lydia E. Pinkham's Vegetable Compound, Dr. Gordon's Elegant Pills, F. J. Kellogg's Safe Fat Reducer*, and *Richard Hudnut's Obesity Pills*, were among scores of pills and potions that invaded the 19th and 20th century marketplaces.

Some culprits even got away with selling arsenic, for use as a digestive remedy, to an ignorant and gullible population. The marketing of nostrums through newspaper advertisements also led to the newspaper market explosion.[3] Even today, pharmaceutical advertisements are the bread-n-butter of periodicals.

A nostrum is a so-called *medicine whose effectiveness is unproved and whose ingredients are usually secret*. We should keep this definition in mind when considering the efficacy of today's pills and potions. Secret ingredients, secured by patents, abound in today's pharmaceutical industry just as it did during the mid-1800s. This is because today's so-called established drug industry is an outgrowth of the patent medicine debacle of previous earlier centuries.

Patented medicines, which numbered nearly 100,000, generated over $3 million dollars in 1859. By 1904, that figure multiplied by ten. Today, pharmaceuticals capture approximately $150 billion annually from consumers.[5] Add other so-called natural remedies to the tab and the figure rises astronomically.

Some of these nostrums caused disappointment because they did not work. Others caused sickness and permanent injury. Still others caused death. The vast incidence of injury, resulting from toxic remedies was one of two urgencies that forced the U.S. government to create the Food and Drug Administration (FDA). The charge of the Agency was to protect citizens against the unscrupulous dealings of nostrum makers and food adulterers.[6] It did this by regulating the process by which medicines are marketed to the public.

Quackery, however, continued to rule the land. Anyone had the opportunity to make and market a concoction that bore false claims. This remains the case today, despite piles of regulatory papers, robust laboratories, and multitudes of investigators. The FDA usually intervenes after the medicines ring up a toll of injury and death. This point must be considered.

For example, the FDA was slow in stopping the marketing of the infamous *Radithor* concoction.[7] This patented medicine goes down as one of the most dangerous in the early history of the FDA. Radithor was radioactive water that contained tiny amounts of radium. It went on sale in 1925. The maker, William J. Bailey, a shady businessman, claimed that the concoction could heal all metabolic disorders. He further boasted that it was harmless. He lied, of course.

Shortly after this nostrum went on sale, reports surfaced about the harm it was causing. It was not until an FDA investigator visited the home of a well-known businessman, who had taken over 1,000 bottles of the drug, and found him wasted away, that the FDA stopped the sale of Radithor. This was in 1931. Between 1925 and 1931, approximately 100,000 bottles a year were sold. This event has been played out repeatedly throughout past decades.

During that time, medicines were assumed safe until proven otherwise. This meant that every medication was granted a cushion of tolerance for causing harm and death. Currently, clinical trials are supposed to ensure that drugs are safe. Yet, drugs have continued to destroy lives despite all the so-called clinical trial phases that accommodate the testing and, subsequent, approval of a drug. Of late, this fact has been confirmed with the banning of an obesity and diabetes drug within the past decade.

People ignorantly assume that an FDA approval of a drug means the drug is safe to use. This is illogical simply on the premise of drug efficacy. The mere fact that every drug comes with a set of adverse reactions indicates that drugs are not safe. Having these negative reactions means that after taking the drug, injury is imminent, severe injury is probable, and death is possible. When it comes to drugs, safety is a notion.

The correlation of this dark period in American history with today's healthcare environment is evident. Let us briefly dissect the prevailing conditions that produced the dietary dark age of the 19th and 20th centuries.

First, eating habits produced digestive disorders, and false dietary advice continued to aggravate them. According to epidemiological studies, several leading chronic diseases that cause high morbidity and mortality are diet-related.[8] These include heart disease, diabetes, and hypertension, to name a few. The impact of these diseases disproportionately affects the poor, just as it did during the 19th century.

And, as the *"belief was widespread that all foods contained one 'universal element' which kept life going, so quantity and not quality was stressed"*, beliefs along that line are the driver behind the chronic disease epidemic. For example, government advises us to eat three or more meals a day. Consequently, overeating or gluttony remains a national habit and digestive-related disorders continue to wreck havoc on the population.

In establishing that the healthcare environment is the same today as it was then, we also confirm that quackery is in full throttle, across the board — in what is termed "quackery" and mainstream, legitimate healthcare. This is according to reality, and the definition of quackery.

The *Online Medical Dictionary*, published by the University of Newcastle upon Tyne in the United Kingdom, defines quackery as:[9]

> *Deliberate misrepresentation of the ability of a substance or device for the prevention or treatment of disease...Quackery also applies to persons who pretend to be able to diagnose or heal people but are unqualified and incompetent.*

Here, rest two major considerations in assessing quackery — 1) the person is unqualified and incompetent to diagnose and heal a patient but pretends to be otherwise, and 2) the person is misrepresenting a substance as a cure or treatment for disease when it is not that. Scanning today's healthcare horizon, we can clearly see that both modes of quackery are pervasive throughout America and the world.

The current state, therefore, is the dietary dark ages of previous centuries multiplied 100 times. Obesity, diabetes, and chronic disease epidemics have worsened and they continue to worsen. No relief of these crises is foreseen. In fact, it is just the opposite — more disease and death.

The formula that disease equals profits also proves the destructive extent of the dietary dark ages. Annual health expenditures account for more than $1.5 trillion.[10] The breakout of this cost is startling. For example, the cost estimate for cardiovascular disease and stroke is $351.8 billion; cancer is $171.6 billion; diabetes is $98 billion; and arthritis is $82 billion.

The growth of disease epidemics corresponds with the growth of healthcare costs, so what are people really getting for their money? And, despite the elaborate show of medical research and technology, the enormity of health studies and reports, clinical trials, drug research, state-of-the-art medical facilities, high-tech medical equipment, medical specialists, herbs, potions, and health legislations, the evidence shows that all of this supports a system of quackery. The evidence is that too few people, if any, are healed of anything through all of this.

In another book by James Harvey Young, *American Health Quackery*, the premise for this deadly ploy is revealed. He writes:[11]

> *...This is possible because the American mind as I have defined it consists of a group of generalizations so sweeping that it is hospitable to different and conflicting particular views.*

Mind, in this context, is the collective conscious and unconscious processes that direct and influence mental and physical behavior. Thinking is among these processes, and the basis of thought is language — words and images arranged and expressed through various ways to represent knowledge.[12]

A primary use of language is to communicate thoughts. Therefore, it is through language that a person's mind is shaped or influenced. A person's concepts, perceptions, dispositions, imagination and ideas are formed through language.

With this in mind, we can conclude that the mathematical precision of one's language ultimately determines the keenest of one's mind.

In the book, *Languages of the Brain*, the editors state:[12]

> *It (language) is used to represent the world and one's interpretation of it; it is used to organize information, to help store information in memory; and to reason about the world and one's place in it.*

Therefore, if language is obscure and confusing, disallowing effective communication and truthful representation of reality, then the person's mental state becomes warped. As a result, a person's entire view of the world, as well as his or her place in it also becomes false. This makes the person a perfect candidate for deception — the greatest of which is to deceive a person into devaluing his or her life.

This deception produces lifestyles, which appear glorifying and productive, but in reality are destructive. Over a course of time, the person views his or her dreadful circumstances as "real" or "keeping it real" when in reality that dreadful *lifestyle* has been manufactured for them by the *merchants of death*.

We must note that other factors also impede our ability to perceive reality properly, such as eating swine flesh. However, language is more effective because it spins a web that captures everyone — swine eater, meat eater, and vegetarian, alike.

Actually, anyone eating swine flesh is a victim of deceptive lingo. This deception has made something unhealthy and deadly seem good to eat. For example, "The Other White Meat" is among the crafty lingo used to promote the consumption of this worm-infested flesh.

In the quote from Mr. Young, the term *sweeping* means that everything, in this world, that affects our lives is mired in generalizations. Confusion abounds. The lines between *fact* and *fiction*, *truth* and *falsehood*, and *yes* and *no* does not exist. Everything is covered in gray. Such a mind operates in shallowness, which makes the frivolous things seem most important, and the principles that govern life, meaningless. Fickleness is the offspring of such nonsense.

Mr. Young further states:

> *People can use the same venerated words with meanings that vary from each other.*

There are scores of definitions for love, happiness, life, liberty, freedom, disease, health and so forth. One man's love is another man's lust. One man's freedom is another man's bondage. Yet, lives are destroyed through misunderstandings, as well as through laws fashioned from such ambiguity. As the cliché goes — ambiguity is the seed of disorder.

And, despite the volumes of laws and law books, disorder and mayhem is pervasive. Few places in the world are without confusion and disorder. The home, school, workshop, city halls, and corporate edifices are ridden with mayhem and confusion.

Divine guidance is absolutely essential, because inherent in such Guidance are the true meanings of these words, and the proper application of them in one's life. Divine instruction leaves no room for guesswork. Human behavior is managed in concert with the mandates of God. This aspect is discussed in Chapter 6.

Another problem is the constant conjuring of words for the express purpose of deceiving the public. Industry leaders continuously add new terms to add ambiguity to reality. For example, consider the concept of "side-effects". This term is used throughout the pharmaceutical and medical industries.

Now, although our everyday living shows that the body operates as a single entity, this fact is not considered when medication is concocted and prescribed. Knowing that the body operates as a single entity, we can surmise that the solution to any disease has a single root. When the root-cause is treated, the body is healed, without producing horrible complications to other areas of the body.

This is not the case with mainstream medicine. We know this. In mainstream medicine, the body is segmented into various parts, with each medical specialist only tending to a specific part. In such an approach, a disease symptom occurring in one part of the body is often treated without any investigation as to the effects the treatment will have on other parts. As a result, when people ingest chemical concoctions to treat one disease symptom, other body organs and functions are negatively affected. Medical professionals called these adverse reactions *side-effects* — a deceptively lighthearted term to describe a physical assault that is really a "risk factor".

A risk factor is something that increases risk or susceptibility to a negative affect or outcome. In medicine, this sometimes is irreversible injury or death.

Therefore, if taking a drug damages other body organs and body functions, then the drug is a risk factor and not a side-effect. Scores of records are available that show the injury and death caused by the so-called side-effects of drugs. To boot, we continuously witness the banning of drugs from the market after they ring up a toll of fatalities.

Capturing these side-effects, in the form of data, has become a booming industry. More money is spent on more foolishness. And, as with most profit-centered industries, this one is corroded with culprits bent on getting around the system. Many incidences of harmful drug reactions go unreported or under-reported. So, drugs that should have been off the market long ago, continue to wreck havoc on patients.[13]

Unfortunately, most people casually accept the "side effects" associated with the nostrums of today's pharmaceutical giants. Ambiguous and deceptive language makes this possible. However, if anyone had to risk losing a right arm to treat a left eye, most of us would reject that treatment. The drug makers, however, do not put the side-effects in this explicit context, although this is precisely where it belongs.

The *merchants of death* usually list a set of seemingly mild discomforts associated with the medication to make these adverse reactions appear inconsequential to one's health. If people viewed these plentiful discomforts correctly, they would realize the serious injury occurring in their bodies. In the end, no healing takes place. The side-effects either exacerbate the initial complaint or produce more severe complaints. Today, most drugs do both.

As insignificant as this observation might appear, it is one of many indicators of the collapse of a civilization. When a society's language gradually becomes imprecise, thus making language the primary vehicle for the delivery of deception and injustice, that society is steeped in darkness and on its way out.

History has revealed obesity to be a long-standing health crisis for profit's sake. Today, this crisis has culminated into national and global pandemics that will continue to wreck havoc on the human family far into the future. Of course, we can avoid this travesty. To do so there must be a national, and then worldwide, agreement on and acceptance of the best diet for humans. This diet is detailed in Chapter 6.

CHAPTER 2

Obesity Crises: Contemporary View

Since the mid-1900's, obesity has been regarded as the number one health problem in Western countries.[14] Its prevalence has also spread to other nations on the earth, making obesity the most urgent global health problem.[15]

In the United States (U.S.), obesity has dramatically risen to epidemic proportions. According to the National Center for Health Statistics, many Americans are overweight and the condition is constantly increasing despite past and current attempts to curtail this epidemic.

Overweight is determined by using the Body Mass Index (BMI) system. BMI is calculated by dividing a person's body weight by their height, squared. Table 1 list the BMI parameters from the National Institutes of Health.

Categorically, a person can have a normal or abnormal BMI. An abnormal BMI is classified as underweight, overweight, and obese. A BMI of 18.5 or below is underweight. Health conditions of underweight persons include fatigued, poor physical stamina and low resistance to infections. Also, health ailments such as tuberculosis, respiratory disorders, pneumonia, circulatory diseases, cerebral hemorrhage, nephritis, and cancer are common among chronically underweight people.

The BMI of normal weight persons is between 20 and 25. This BMI is associated with low health risks and low premature death rates, as compared to overweight or obese persons. A BMI between 25 and 30 is classified as overweight, and a BMI over 30 puts the person in the obesity category. These two categories are associated with increased risk for many major chronic diseases that lead to early mortality.

Recent data indicate that approximately 64% of American adults are either overweight or obese.[16] This is up from 55% in 1994, and reflects a doubling in the rate of overweight since 1980.[17] Some surveys indicate that 74% of Americans are overweight.[18]

When statisticians render these figures, they fail to mention that approximately 226 million people live in the U.S. The situation suddenly becomes more alarming. For example, there are 129.6 million adults (20+ years old) overweight, of which 64.5 million are women and 65.1 million are men, comprising 61.9% and 67.2%, respectively.[16] The nearly one-third of U.S. adults who are obese equates to 61.3 million (30.5%), of which 34.7 million (33.4%) are women and 26.6 million (27.5%) are men.

Table 1: Body Mass Index Table

BMI	19	20	21	22	23	24	25	26	27	28	29	30	31	32	33	34	35
Hgt. (inch)	Body Weight (pounds)																
58	91	96	100	105	110	115	119	124	129	134	138	143	148	153	158	162	167
59	94	99	104	109	114	119	124	128	133	138	143	148	153	158	163	168	173
60	97	102	107	112	118	123	128	133	138	143	148	153	158	163	168	174	179
61	100	106	111	116	122	127	132	137	143	148	153	158	164	169	174	180	185
62	104	109	115	120	126	131	136	142	147	153	158	164	169	175	180	186	191
63	107	113	118	124	130	135	141	146	152	158	163	169	175	180	186	191	197
64	110	116	122	128	134	140	145	151	157	163	169	174	180	186	192	197	204
65	114	120	126	132	138	144	150	156	162	168	174	180	186	192	198	204	210
66	118	124	130	136	142	148	155	161	167	173	179	186	192	198	204	210	216
67	121	127	134	140	146	153	159	166	172	178	185	191	198	204	211	217	223
68	125	131	138	144	151	158	164	171	177	184	190	197	203	210	216	223	230
69	128	135	142	149	155	162	169	176	182	189	196	203	209	216	223	230	236
70	132	139	146	153	160	167	174	181	188	195	202	209	216	222	229	236	243
71	136	143	150	157	165	172	179	186	193	200	208	215	222	229	236	243	250
72	140	147	154	162	169	177	184	191	199	206	213	221	228	235	242	250	258
73	144	151	159	166	174	182	189	197	204	212	219	227	235	242	250	257	265
74	148	155	163	171	179	186	194	202	210	218	225	233	241	249	256	264	272
75	152	160	168	176	184	192	200	208	216	224	232	240	248	256	264	272	279
76	156	164	172	180	189	197	205	213	221	230	238	246	254	263	271	279	287
From National Institutes of Health, National Heart, Blood, and Lung Institute																	

Equally as serious a problem is the epidemic of "super-obesity" or "morbid obesity". An analysis of increases in obesity from 1986 to 2000 showed that the percentage increase of the heaviest Americans has grown faster than obesity itself. Over this period, those with a BMI of 30 or more increased by about 80%; those with a BMI of 40 by 350%, and those with a BMI of 50 or more by 500%.[19]

Epidemiological data also shows the prevalence of obesity in specific populations. For example, the age-adjusted prevalence of combined overweight and obesity in racial/ethnic groups is as follows:[20]

- 77.3% of Non-Hispanic Black women
- 71.9% of Mexican American women
- 57.3% of Non-Hispanic White women
- 60.7% of Non-Hispanic Black men
- 74.7% of Mexican American men
- 67.4% of Non-Hispanic White men

Overall, studies indicate that those with children, Black people, women, those with a lower education level, those from the Midwest, and those who have a lower level of physical activity during leisure time are more likely to be obese than others.[21] These "others" must be the one or two persons left, as most people meet one or more of the above characteristics.

Childhood Obesity

Another grave consideration is the rise in obesity among children. In the U.S., childhood obesity has now been identified as a major threat to children's health.[22] According to some reports, 13% of children ages 6 to 11 years, and 14% of adolescents ages 12 to 19 years are overweight.[23] This prevalence has nearly tripled for adolescents in the past two decades. The rise in obesity among children mirrored that of adults, indicating that America's families are generally overweight. The lack of physical activity is among several factors causing the epidemic in childhood obesity.

The epidemic of childhood obesity presents two important concerns. The first concern is the short-term health consequences. The most common set of ailments found in obese or overweight children are hypertension, dyslipidemia and psychosocial problems.[24]

Obese children also experience orthopedic, neurologic, pulmonary, gastroenterologic, endocrinologic, metabolic, and cardiovascular disorders.[25] Approximately 60% of overweight children have developed at least one cardiovascular risk factor (i.e. high blood pressure, lipid levels or impaired glucose tolerance) and 20% of overweight children have two or more of these.[26]

The secondary, but equally as important concern, is the child-obesity/adult-obesity link. The persistence of obesity into the adult years is associated with increased risk and incidence of adult cardiovascular morbidity and mortality.[27]

Overall, the increase in childhood obesity means that, in the coming decades, we can expect increases in adult obesity and its related diseases. This reality significantly affects current attempts to curb healthcare costs, for unless childhood obesity is reduced, annual healthcare expenditures will continue to soar.[24]

Around the World

As previously addressed, the global population has succumbed to obesity. According to the World Health Organization (WHO), obesity is a global pandemic — the most recent estimates being that a billion people are overweight and 300 million are obese.[28]

WHO pins the rising epidemic to profound changes in society and in the behavioral patterns of communities over recent decades. For example, economic growth, modernization, urbanization and globalization of food markets are among the forces driving the obesity pandemic. Diets with a higher proportion of fats, saturated fats and sugars have supplemented urban wholesome diets.

Additionally, societal shifts in away from occupations that require more physical and mental activity play major roles in the rise of obesity. For example, in some countries, there is less physically demanding work. This, combined with increased uses of automated transportation systems and home technologies, has reduced physical demands.

Other researchers attribute the obesity pandemic to the spread of Westernization to other countries.[29] In addition to so-called democracy, Westernization features fast foods and a sedentary lifestyle.

Obesity Definition and Classification

Perhaps among the many things that have convoluted the obesity crisis is how to define and classify the condition. Here, we examine these two issues.

Definition

Tom Brody, in the book, *Nutritional Biochemistry*, presents a solid definition of obesity.[30] He writes:

> *Obesity can be defined as a process where fat accumulates over a long period of time due to an increased rate of storage of triglycerides in adipose tissue...a plateau of weight is finally reached where the percentage of body fat is maintained, and where any attempt to lose weight is resisted by a powerful drive to return to the weight plateau.*

This definition provides several insights. One is the duration of obesity. As most people know, this condition does not come about instantaneously. The long duration in the development of obesity points to an abnormal alteration in metabolism. Therefore, some researchers have called obesity a metabolic disorder. This has merit.

Metabolism is the sum total of all the chemical reactions occurring in the body cells. Essentially, this is the breaking down and building up of substances that support the life of the cell, which is the basic physiological unit of life. These reactions transform substances into energy or materials the cells require.

There is more to this, but suffice it to say, this natural and life-supporting activity must be sustained, in balance. The body needs what it needs, and having any more or any less than what it needs, potentially, causes the body to malfunction. Imbalance occurs. This condition is either temporary or long-termed.

Obesity is a chronic imbalance that gradually registers as life-threatening, as the body takes on a new form — deformity. In one sense, this phenomenon is awesome, as it shows why human life is the most magnificent life form. Our ability to adapt is incredible.

It demonstrates our superiority over other creatures and over creation. However, in another sense, this remarkable ability has the potential to destroy us. Obesity is perhaps the clearest demonstration of the destructive power of adaptability.

Another insight in Mr. Brody's definition of obesity is that of "plateau". This means that certain thresholds of fat accumulation are crossed. Once this happens, attempts to return to one's normal and balanced conditions become difficult. This is not to imply that such a goal is impossible to achieve. However, this effort may be as long in duration as it took to accumulate the excess fat. People have to understand this when seeking treatment. They have to be prepared for the long haul back to normal weight.

Classification

Again, controversies yet persist about how to classify obesity. Some health researchers have termed it a disease, while others have called it a biological adaptation.[31] Of late, the term "genetic disorder" has surfaced.[32] Scientists hypothesize that an obesity gene exists. This is highly debatable, and in some instances, outlandish.

Medical professionals agree that there is a genetic predisposition to obesity, as it is with many other diseases. This is not a grand revelation. This is natural to life itself, as we pass our genes to our offspring. Our genetic makeup is contained in the life germ.

At best, this means that our immediate offspring may possess the potential to develop the metabolic-related health ailments we encountered, just as they have the potential to develop the good traits — intelligence, musical or artistic inclination, and so forth — that we, as parents, have.

This, of course, does not necessarily guarantee that they will develop any of these things, good or bad. If their artistic potential is tapped through desire and proper instruction, they can equal or better their parents in that ability. Just the same, if they eat the same poor quality foods as their parents, then ill-health and obesity will be their lot. If they eat better, then they will live healthier and longer than did their parents.

The latter is the most certain aspect about obesity or overweight — its connection with food. Without food, no one could become overweight. There are, of course, other factors besides the over consumption of food that assist with causing obesity. Among these are the types and biochemical qualities of the foods ingested, and how frequently these foods are eaten.

The World Health Organization's position on obesity supports its association with diet. WHO states:

More often than not, obesity is the result of unhealthy eating habits coupled with a sedentary way of life...Energy storage is part of the body's natural protection against famine and is fundamental for survival when food is scarce. However, when energy storage becomes the rule rather than the exception, it leads to obesity...

This means that obesity has a "self-induced" component. Medical researchers' and pharmaceutical companies' persistence to label obesity a disease is deceptive. This position rolls out the carpet for the spewing of toxic pills and potions into the marketplace, as it takes away from us the authority to control the causes of this condition. This false disposition also encourages us to blame everyone else but ourselves for our own ill-health.

If researchers persist in seeking a disease classification for obesity, then the best arena for such classification is "mental" disease. In this sense, it is mental disease that results from misinformation, deception, and a lack of proper education about the human body and how best to sustain it. Therefore, medication to address this disease is not a pill or elixir, but it is truth and proper education.

Biology of Weight Gain

The pathology of obesity is a major research objective in mainstream medical research.[33] This is because the biology of weight gain is the biology of disease acquisition, as some major chronic diseases are acquired through weight gain. Again, obesity in its simplest definition is inordinate body fat mass.

Health researchers have long known that excess fat, or in the scientific term, excessive *adipose tissue*, is associated with a number of chronic diseases — hyperlipidaemia, high blood pressure, carbohydrate intolerance and diabetes, coronary atherosclerotic heart disease, gout, restrictive lung disease, gall bladder disease, cancer, degenerative arthritis, and infertility, to name a few.[34] This is why weight reduction is the only sound and proven intervention for obesity-related chronic diseases.[35] The central or worldwide debate is how best to achieve and sustain healthy weight.

The adipose or fat cell is a primary player in the biology of weight gain. The biological workings of this cell are very interesting and knowledge of its workings in storing excessive fat should fortify our resolve to accept the best diet for humans, once that diet has been clearly delineated. This delineation is presented in Chapter 6.

Here, it is appropriate to state that all the cells in the body are specialized to perform particular functions. This is very fascinating because the body starts out as a single cell, which multiplies millions of times, while producing many types of different looking, as well as diverse, functioning cells.

Adipose cells serve one primary purpose and that is to store excess nutrients as fat. This tissue is present in all mammalian species, as all mammalian species, at one point or another, have need to adapt to environmental conditions that require the storage of fat or use of fat stores.

In understanding adipose tissue, scientists have categorized this tissue according to its two general functions — store fat and produce heat. Adipose tissue that store fat is called *white* fat; and fat used for heat production is termed *brown* fat. Obesity concerns primarily white fat.

Figure 1. Portal Venous System

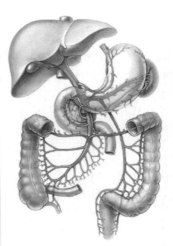

There are many unique features about white adipose tissue in comparison with other body cells. One feature is that it can markedly change its mass after adult size is reached. Fat mass can range from 2% - 70% of body weight. The latter is the percentage associated with massively obese persons.

Adipose tissue is found throughout the body, as fat depots are located in the upper and lower body regions. For example, a few of these areas include the neck, shoulders, chest, abdomen, hips, breast and thighs. Most people inspect one or more of these areas to determine if they have gained weight.

Generally, the fat deposits are classified as subcutaneous or visceral. Subcutaneous is the fat tissue layered under the skin.

Visceral is the fat accumulated in the abdominal area. Excess fat in this area is called central obesity, and poses a greater risk of disease.

Fat accumulation in the visceral area, in association with the portal venous system, exposes the liver to the polluted substances secreted by these fat depots.[36] The increase in adipose tissue means the release of more free fatty acids, glycerol, and lactate — all of which injures the internal digestive organs, especially the liver.

The pathology of obesity involves the response of adipose tissue to the demand made upon it to store excessive fat, in the form of triglycerides. This demand forces it to either increase the size of adipocytes or fat cells, or produce more fat cells. Scientifically, these responses are called cellular *hypertrophy* (increase in size) and *hyperplasia* (increase in number), respectively.[37]

Studies in humans and non-humans, alike, indicate that the increase in cell size precedes the increase in cell number.[38] In more simplistic lingo, once the current cells "max out" in their ability to handle the storage demands, the body mechanisms signal for the production of more cells.

Again, the fat cell is, specifically, designed to store energy as fat, so it does this whether it has to expand to the limit or produce additional cells to handle the load. This biological adaptation is on automatic pilot, meaning it does not require our conscious approval to perform this task.

Consequently, this hyperplastic condition is associated with the most severe forms of obesity.[39] It also makes for the poorest prognosis for treatment.[40] This is because the body has crossed a threshold wherein the reversibility of this condition becomes extremely formidable. Crossing this threshold means a person has entered the "super" or "morbid" obesity realm — for after the body signals the adipose tissue to begin producing additional cells to meet the storage demand, at what point does it signal the body to shut it off?

The assumed answer is when there is no need for additional cells to store fat. However, the expansion of this tissue invokes neuronal and hormonal processes that make it hard to push the breakfast, lunch, and dinner plates away. Also, the potential to regain the weight hovers over the person like a dark cloud. Albeit, all is not lost. In adopting the best lifestyle change, which includes proper diet, people are able to make calculable improvements in weight loss and overall health.

Obesity: An Enemy Of Life

The Honorable Louis Farrakhan takes us through the complications of obesity in his book, *A Torchlight For America*:[41]

The first casualty of FAT is the physical appearance, which it utterly destroys. It literally distorts the human form, leaving almost no area of the body untouched. It makes a home in the face, the jaws, the chin, neck, upper back, lower back, arms... — wherever it can find a resting place, it settles and cripples the useful muscles and organs of the body.

This unnecessary, unwanted, excess fat gathers around the veins and arteries. It also clogs the veins and arteries, making it difficult for the blood to flow...To meet the increased workload, the heart may add muscle fibers, which places an additional burden on it until it is simply unable to continue and fails.

The medical equation for this grave condition is:

Obesity = increased morbidity and increased mortality

The health consequences associated with obesity are enormous, as it is the greatest risk factor for nearly every chronic disease that leads to morbidity and early death. According to one report, the death rate of obese persons reflects a greater susceptibility to degenerative disease, *"notably diabetes, cirrhosis of the liver, and heart, kidney and circulatory diseases."* Obesity increases the risk of death from cardiovascular and kidney diseases by more than 50%.[42]

Overweight and obese persons show a greater than normal mortality rate, and this rate increases with the degree of obesity. For example, death among moderately obese men is 42% above the standard risk, and among the markedly obese, 79% above. Generally, obese persons age 20-44 have a 3.8 times greater risk of type II diabetes, 5.6 times greater risk of hypertension, and 2.1 times greater risk of hypercholesterolemia.

Obesity also brings about increased mortality from all cancers. The incidence rates of several types of cancer are elevated in overweight individuals. These include cancer of the colon, rectum, and prostate in men; and uterus, biliary tract, breast, and ovary in women.

The detrimental effects of obesity do not stop there. Obesity has been linked to enlarged hearts[43] and is also associated with sleep disruption conditions, such as asthma, gastroesophageal reflux, sleep apnea, and nocturia.[44]

A variety of other medical disorders is associated with obesity. These include degenerative joint disease (both weight bearing and non-weight bearing joints), diseases of the digestive tract (gallstones, reflux esophagitis), thromboembolic disorders, heart failure, respiratory impairment, and skin disorders. Obese persons have a greater incidence of surgical and obstetric complications and are more prone to accidents. Also, obese patients are at risk of psychological disorders and social discrimination.

Table 2 lists the physical ailments associated with overweight and obesity.

Table 2: Obesity-Related Complications

Arthritis	Osteoarthritis of knee and hip
Rheumatoid arthritis	Birth Defects
Cancers	Breast Cancer in Women
Breast Cancer in Men	Cancers of the Esophagus and Gastric Cardia
Colorectal Cancer	Endometrial Cancer
Renal Cell Cancer	Cardiovascular Disease
Carpal Tunnel Syndrome	Chronic Venous Insufficiency
Daytime Sleepiness	Deep Vein Thrombosis
End Stage Renal Disease	Gallbladder Disease
Gout	Heart Disorders
Hypertension	Impaired Immune Response
Impaired Respiratory Function	Infections Following Wounds
Infertility	Liver Disease
Low Back Pain	Obstetric and Gynecological Complications
Pain	Severe Acute Biliary and Alcoholic Pancreatitis
Sleep Apnea	Stroke
Surgical Complications	Traumatic Injuries to Teeth
Type 2 Diabetes (NIDDM)	Urinary Stress Incontinence

Of late, scientists have assembled obesity-related ailments into a sort of disease gumbo. They call it *metabolic syndrome X*. Perhaps this is a legitimate effort to provide more responsive treatment, or a greater ploy to gain more money by confusing the issue. Regardless to which it is, this approach is not new.

In 1933, the clustering of hypertension, obesity and gout were grouped as an X syndrome.[45] Thereafter, medical scientists conjured several other names, including *insulin resistance syndrome, cardiovascular metabolic syndrome,* and *the deadly quartet.* The concept of syndrome X for the clustering of cardiovascular risk factors — hypertension, obesity, high triglyceride and low HDL cholesterol concentrations — was re-introduced in the late 1980s.

In 1998, WHO proposed a definition for metabolic syndrome — *patients with type 2 diabetes mellitus or impaired glucose tolerance have the syndrome if they have two or more of the following ailments: microalbuminuria, hypertension, dyslipidemia, and obesity.* Regardless to the name, weight loss has been found to reduce metabolic syndrome,[46] just as it is key to reducing obesity and diabetes risks and related-diseases. We reiterate that the key issue is how this weight is reduced.=

Quality of Life

Biomechanical Difficulties

The Honorable Louis Farrakhan writes in the *Final Call Newspaper*:

> *We have overburdened our skeletal muscles with unwanted FAT. Bone, muscle, tendon and ligament are designed to work together in a harmonious relationship to move the body. When we stand, our entire weight is carried by the power of our legs down to our feet. If taxed by excess weight, muscle wears down and eventually falters.*

Now, numerous studies have surfaced, providing greater information about the affect of excessive poundage on the human vessel. For example, studies have shown that high levels of body fat, plus increased loads on the major joints have the potential to lead to pain and discomfort, inefficient body mechanics and further reductions in mobility.[47]

Other research has entertained the challenges faced by overweight and obese persons in completing simple daily activities, such as walking. For example, the feet, as the base of support of the body, are continually exposed to high ground reaction forces generated during activities of daily living. Excessive increases in weight-bearing force caused by obesity are detrimental to the lower limbs and feet.[47]

Minister Farrakhan continues:

There is a precise, mathematical relationship between skeleton, height and weight. Like the bones, the skeletal muscle range in size and shape to suit the particular functions they perform. Their ability to perform with speed and power can be literally of life-or-death importance, enabling us to move in response to sudden danger. When it is not overburdened, skeletal muscle can move into action within a few hundredths of a second and, when necessary, support 1,000 times its own weight.

This "high science" deserves careful study, because it is the science of and about the human being, and touches upon the importance of the mathematical design of the human body in relation to its function. The mathematical relationship between height, weight, and skeleton has not been thoroughly addressed in mainstream health research. Certainly, those who are overweight know that they have become less mobile with the added weight, bearing witness that flexibility, speed, and agility are compromised with the additional weight.

Regarding the *ability to perform with speed and power in life-or-death situations*, we need only consider the number of household and automobile accidents that may be attributed to obesity or overweight. This aspect is not factored into the obesity-health cost burden, nor is it factored into the remedy for preventing unnecessary household and automobile accidents. Lawmakers and insurance companies probably have never considered this specific aspect. This should be considered, especially with more than one-third of the U.S. adult population overweight.

For example, how many obese persons drive cars? In 2000, there were over 6 million automobile accidents — 6,394,000 to be more precise.[48] How many of these accidents involved overweight persons?

Everyone knows that both alertness and the ability to quickly react are very important on today's highways. And, now with increasing speed limits up to 75 miles per hour on some highways, impeccable control of one's automobile is a necessity. Not only does a person have to be quick on the breaks or the gas pedal, but that person must be able to maneuver to avoid collisions. A fat and heavy arm, attached to a huge overweight body, offers very little chance of having such control. This is real.

Therefore, it is not unreasonable to assume that lethargic drivers dominate the highways of America. Not only are such drivers lethargic due to overweight, but also their minds are bogged down with the residue of toxins caused by the constant consumption of food. This makes their thinking slow, as the blood supply is polluted with toxins and the body's energies are constantly concentrated in the digestive process. Drowsiness, therefore, is constantly upon them. They are actually sleeping behind the wheel, despite the fact that their eyes are open.

So, automobile accidents take the lives of many people each year, In addition, it registers substantial economic tolls, such as the toll incurred from loss productivity due to disabilities; the toll on the insurance industry; and the overall burden put on the American taxpayers to foot these losses. A deeper study on obesity will prove that it is, indeed, an enemy to life in many ways not yet considered.

As for the overweight or obese person, the added weight must be viewed as a risk factor for accidents, particularly automobile accidents. This fact should serve as a motivating force to remedy obesity and overweight.

Patient's Perceptions

In health research, healthcare practitioners have mainly focused on clinical data to assess the impact of disease on health and life expectancy. Over the years, it has become increasingly important to measure the impact of disease on a person's quality of life. There is a growing understanding that quality of life is very important to patients and underpins their involvement with the healthcare system.

Quality of life is measured by assessing a patient's feelings or perceptions about the disease and their treatment in the healthcare system. This disposition is far overdue. In the evolution of Western medicine during the last century, the humanity of the patient was not considered. The primary goals were often to test new medication on patients, and to drive up costs by using unnecessary surgical procedures, or other bestial medical practices. The patient was only a number — similar to mice and other lower-creatures used in scientific studies.

Consequently, practitioners and researchers were indifferent to a patient's feelings, well-being or the well-being of the patient's family. Arrogance among medical practitioners was pervasive. This mentality remains when it comes to the treatment of so-called minorities, including women. The appearance and feeling of "apathetic experimentation" is ever-present throughout the healthcare industry.

The concept of health-related quality of life or HRQOL refers to a person or group's perceived physical and mental health, as assessed over a period of time. Generally, HRQOL often includes measurements of physical and social function, psychological status, functional capacity, somatic sensation and the sense of well-being as impacted by health status. Although this data is subjective and difficult to define and measure, HRQOL protocols have made it possible to gather and identify consistent factors that impact quality of life in specific subgroups. Additionally, tracking health-related quality of life in different populations can help guide policies or interventions to improve healthcare delivery.

No doubt, there are quality of life issues with respect to obesity treatment because losing weight is challenging, and the means by which this is done can significantly impact the quality of life of the person suffering obesity or overweight. Much of what is known about quality of life in overweight conditions has been derived from studying obese persons in treatment settings, rather than studying them in a broad range of social and functional settings. Additionally, much of the early research on quality of life and obesity is limited to persons undergoing surgical intervention.

Both physical functioning and psychosocial functioning are negatively impacted by excess weight, with greater impairments associated with greater degrees of obesity.[49] After weight loss, health-related quality of life improves, significantly — even with small to moderate weight loss. The benefits of dramatic weight losses are significantly positive, and these benefits continue for a number of years.[50]

Numerous studies have shown that the heavier a person was in middle-age years, the worse was their perception of the quality of life in old age. In one study, approximately 6,800 people in Chicago had their body-mass index (BMI) calculated when they were between 36 and 64 years of age.[51] Twenty-six years later, they answered 12 questions about their perceived physical and mental conditions. In every category, those with normal BMI had significantly better scores than overweight or obese persons.

Overweight people had more physical limitations, more pain, less energy and reported less social functioning and worse mental health. This study confirmed the obvious — excess weight decreases the quality of life.

In another study, researchers compared the health-related quality of life of overweight and obese persons from different subgroups that vary in *treatment-seeking status* and *treatment intensity*.[52] Participants were from five distinct groups, representing a continuum of treatment intensity: 1) overweight/obese community volunteers who were not enrolled in weight-loss treatment, 2) clinical trial participants, 3) outpatient weight-loss programs/studies participants, 4) participants in a day-treatment program for obesity, and 5) gastric bypass patients.

The results indicated that obesity-specific HRQOL was significantly more impaired in the treatment-seeking groups than in the nontreatment-seeking group across comparable gender and body mass index (BMI) categories. Within the treatment groups, HRQOL varied by treatment intensity. Gastric bypass patients had the most impairment, followed by day-treatment patients, followed by participants in outpatient weight loss programs/studies, followed by participants in clinical trials. Obesity-specific HRQOL was more impaired for those with higher BMIs, and for women in certain treatment groups.

This research points to two key factors. First, seeking treatment for obesity or any health condition is burdensome. Therefore, some persons decide not to receive treatment because it interrupts their normal schedule. This is a mistake because every health condition should be treated.

Seeking and receiving treatment requires modifications to one's usual or normal day-to-day activities. At first, this may seem to be more of a hindrance than a benefit. However, with consistency, the treatment regimen will become a normal part of the person's daily living. This leads to the second factor.

Treatment, when it is a lifestyle change, is best. For example, gradually changing one's diet for the betterment is far less bothersome and burdensome than having to adapt one's lifestyle because of the consequences of bariatric surgery. This issue is addressed in Chapter 5.

CHAPTER 3

Diabetes: The Curable Disease

Diabetes mellitus is a metabolic condition characterized by hyperglycemia — the presence of an abnormally high concentration of glucose in the blood. There are instances throughout the day, particularly when a food or drink that has a high sugar-content is consumed, that the blood-glucose level may be raised beyond normal. However, diabetes is the long-term inability of the body to bring the high blood-glucose level to normal. It is a chronic disease, wherein the body must contend with unfavorable conditions on a continuous basis.

Perhaps, the simplest way to understand diabetes is to see it as a disruption of an essential biofeedback system — a system that is designed to keep the body in proper biological balance. There are many biofeedback mechanisms at work in the body. For example, biofeedback mechanisms control body temperature, regulate heart rate, blood pressure, and blood levels of oxygen, carbon dioxide, and minerals. All biofeedback mechanisms have the primary goal of preventing sudden and severe changes within the body, which could cause disease or death.

It is essential for the body to regulate glucose levels. If the glucose concentration is too low, neural function becomes impaired, leading to adverse health conditions, including comatose. On the other hand, if the glucose concentration is too high, as with diabetes, the condition produces a toxicity that gradually destroys the body, while disrupting other biofeedback systems that depend on the blood-glucose biofeedback mechanism.

All biofeedback mechanisms are interrelated, so a disruption of one usually causes disruptions in others. This is why some diseases are also risk factors for other diseases. Diabetes is a risk factor for heart disease, which is also connected to a biofeedback mechanism, specifically the one that manages blood-lipid levels.

The pancreas is intricately involved with glucose regulation, as it serves an endocrine function by producing the hormones, insulin and glucagon. Both hormones help to regulate the amount of sugar in the blood. Insulin is the chief digestive hormone that regulates sugar uptake in the body. Body cells depend on glucose to carry out vital metabolic functions, so without insulin, body cells are unable to obtain and use glucose.

Figure 2. Pancreas (anterior view)

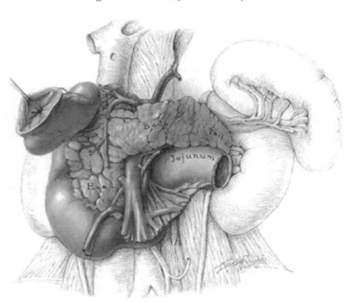

When a person eats a meal, the pancreas is informed by neural signals released from both the central nervous system and intestine. These signals sensitize the pancreas' beta cells so that when the nutrients, including glucose and fat, are absorbed from the intestine, causing an increase in blood-glucose concentration, as well as other blood-nutrient levels, the beta cells respond by secreting insulin.

When insulin is secreted into the blood stream, glucose is taken up by most body cells, and the excess is stored as glycogen in the liver and muscles. Insulin decreases blood-glucose levels by allowing the body to uptake and use the glucose. The action of insulin brings blood sugar levels back to normal. This biofeedback process restores the glucose balance of the body.

Without insulin, glucose builds up in the blood, while the cells and tissues literally starve to death. This causes the blood to become toxic. Tissue degeneration begins to occur. Deficient insulin action on target tissues also causes abnormalities in carbohydrate, fat, and protein metabolism. Scientists believe that glycation of tissue proteins and other macromolecules, and excess production of polyol compounds from glucose are among several mechanisms that damage tissues.

Diabetes Types

Categorically, diabetes is of several types, with the two major being type 1 and type 2. Type 1 is an autoimmune disease, which causes the destruction of the insulin-producing cells of the pancreas. As a result, either no insulin or an insufficient amount of insulin is produced. People with this type of diabetes must take medicinal insulin.

Type 2 diabetes is also called non-insulin-dependent diabetes mellitus (NIDDM) or adult-onset diabetes. Medical scientists believe that this condition is caused by tissue resistance to insulin action and/or an insufficient production of insulin from the pancreas. The mechanisms behind it are still under investigation, however, most everyone agrees that this disease is diet-related.

With respect to obesity's effect on diabetes, some health researchers propose that the permanent elevation of plasma free fatty acids and the predominant use of lipids by the cells impede glucose uptake by the cells, thereby, causing insulin resistance.[53] The rise in insulin secretion is a biofeedback or compensatory mechanism that responds to the increased levels of circulating glucose.

Epidemic Status

Type 2 diabetes is epidemic in the United States. It accounts for approximately 90% of all diagnosed cases of diabetes. Approximately 16 million persons have diabetes, with about 5 million having the disease but not knowing it. Nearly 800,000 new cases of diabetes are diagnosed each year.[54] People, age 65 years or older, account for almost 40% of all diabetics, as aging is a risk factor for the disease.

Obesity is the foremost risk factor, as overeating and overweight are risk factors for type 2 diabetes.[55] For example, the risk for diabetes is two-fold in the mildly obese, five-fold in moderately obese and ten-fold in severely obese persons.[52] Other risk factors include family history of diabetes, prior history of gestational diabetes, impaired glucose tolerance, and physical inactivity.

Figure 3. Pancreas (posterior view)

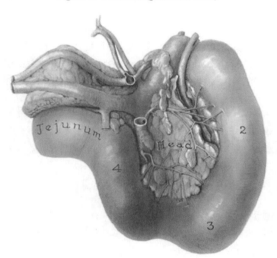

As with obesity, trends show that diabetes disproportionately affect minority populations. Between 1980 and 2000, the age-adjusted prevalence of diagnosed diabetes was higher among Blacks than Caucasians, with Black females having the highest rates. Between 1997 and 2000, the age-adjusted prevalence of diabetes for Hispanic males and females was similar to that of Black males.

Type 2 diabetes among children is epidemic.[57] Once upon a time, it was rare for pediatric centers to have patients with type 2 diabetes. However, by 1994, approximately 16% of new cases of diabetes were among children, particularly those living in urban areas.[58] By 1999, depending on geographic location, the range of percent of new cases rose as much as 45%.[59] The highest incidences of childhood and adolescent diabetes cases were among Blacks,

Mexican Americans, Native Americans and Asian Americans — the same as with obesity.

Globally, diabetes is pandemic, capturing both so-called developing and developed countries. The World Health Organization (WHO) predicts a 170% increase in diabetes in developing countries, and a 42% rise in industrialized countries. We can take from this that not only is diabetes increasing at alarming rates, but also its pandemic nature means that the quality of life of both high-tech and low-tech countries is jeopardized.

Symptoms

At earlier stages, type 2 diabetes is usually not severe enough for people to notice any of the classic symptoms. This form of diabetes usually goes undiagnosed for many years because the hyperglycemia develops gradually.[55] Symptoms of marked hyperglycemia include *polyuria*, *polydipsia*, weight loss, sometimes with *polyphagia*, and blurred vision.

In polyuria, the excessive glucose in the kidney filtrate acts as an osmotic diuretic, inhibiting water resorption by the kidney tubules. This causes a huge urine output that leads to decreased blood volume.

Many electrolytes are lost during polyuria. This causes mineral imbalance. It also results in dehydration, which stimulates hypothalamic thirst centers; thus causing polydipsia, or excessive thirst.

Additionally, there is an excessively abnormal hunger for food, called polyphagia. This biological response is caused by the absence of satiety that is usually experienced when glucose enters the cells. The diabetic must overcome strong metabolically-induced cravings to eat sugar-filled foods.

Health Consequences

Diabetes is a dreaded disease. Generally, the health consequence of this condition is the discombobulating of the human vessel. There is a gradually painful dismantling of all body organs and functions. The chronic hyperglycemia of diabetes is associated with the long-term failure of various organs, especially the eyes, kidneys, nerves, heart, and blood vessels. The person with this disease literally falls to pieces. The emotional and social impact of diabetes, and the demands of therapy also cause significant psychosocial dysfunction in patients and their families. Table 3 describes the complications associated with diabetes.[60]

Table 3: Complications of Diabetes

Complication	Epidemiological Stature
Heart Disease	• Heart disease is the leading cause of diabetes-related deaths. Adults with diabetes have heart disease death rates about 2 to 4 times higher than adults without diabetes. • The risk for stroke is 2 to 4 times higher among people with diabetes. • About 65% of deaths among people with diabetes are due to heart disease and stroke.
High Blood Pressure	• About 73% of adults with diabetes have blood pressure greater than or equal to 130/80 mm Hg or use prescription medications for hypertension.
Blindness	• Diabetes is the leading cause of new cases of blindness among adults aged 20-74 years. • Diabetic retinopathy causes 12,000 to 24,000 new cases of blindness each year.
Kidney Disease	• Diabetes is the leading cause of end-stage renal disease, accounting for 44 percent of new cases. • In 2001, 42,813 people with diabetes began treatment for end-stage renal disease. • In 2001, a total of 142,963 people with end-stage renal disease due to diabetes were living on chronic dialysis or with a kidney transplant.
Nervous System Disease	• About 60% to 70% of people with diabetes have mild to severe forms of nervous system damage. The results of such damage include impaired sensation or pain in the feet or hands, slowed digestion of food in the stomach, carpal tunnel syndrome, and other nerve problems. • Severe forms of diabetic nerve disease are a major contributing cause of lower-extremity amputations.
Amputations	• More than 60% of nontraumatic lower-limb amputations occur among people with diabetes. • In 2000-2001, about 82,000 nontraumatic lower-limb amputations were performed annually among people with diabetes.
Dental Disease	• Periodontal (gum) disease is more common among people with diabetes. Among young adults, those with diabetes have about twice the risk of those without diabetes. • Almost one-third of people with diabetes have severe periodontal diseases with loss of attachment of the gums to the teeth measuring 5 millimeters or more.
Complications of pregnancy	• Poorly controlled diabetes before conception and during the first trimester of pregnancy can cause major birth defects in 5% to 10% of pregnancies and spontaneous abortions in 15% to 20% of pregnancies. • Poorly controlled diabetes during the second and third trimesters of pregnancy can result in excessively large babies, posing a risk to the mother and the child.
Other Complications	• Uncontrolled diabetes often leads to biochemical imbalances that can cause acute life-threatening events, such as diabetic ketoacidosis and hyperosmolar (nonketotic) coma. • People with diabetes are more susceptible to many other illnesses and, once they acquire these illnesses, often have worse prognoses. For example, they are more likely to die with pneumonia or influenza than people who do not have diabetes.

Solution

Now that we know what diabetes is and the disastrous health conditions associated with it, the most important concern is *how to prevent and cure this condition*. Type 2 diabetes, as a dietary-related disease, means that the first line of defense — prevention and intervention — is to adopt a dietary practice that eliminates and prevents this dreaded condition.

With respect to the *diabetes-obesity* connection, studies have shown that weight loss reduces this condition.[61] This is logical, as weight loss improves all obesity-related ailments. However, how the weight is reduced is as equally as important, especially where the use of weight-reducing concoctions are concerned. For example, the probability that the popular quack nostrum, Metabolife, might have been linked to the development of diabetic ketoacidosis, prompt scientific investigations.[62] Hopefully, people are learning that quick fixes to metabolic disorders are recipes for disaster.

Additionally certain low-fat food products increase diabetes risk. For example, studies have shown that trans-fatty acids, which comprise margarine and other butter substitutes, increase the risk of diabetes.[63]

As we have learned and will continue to address (in the upcoming chapters), weight loss as a main goal is inadequate in bringing about complete health restoration. Weight loss should not be the core objective of obesity or diabetes treatments. When weight loss is the primary aim, a person is easily fooled into ingesting toxic pills or consuming unhealthy, highly toxic foods and drinks, masked as health-oriented remedies. This, again, is sheer quackery.

When the real treatment for obesity and diabetes is applied or practiced, weight loss is achieved. Weight loss should be the natural result of a healthy way of living, which includes a dietary practice that has longevity as its goal. And, in the context of this book, longevity is not the meager 55, 60, or 65 years many people live today. It is beyond these. The connection of diet to longevity is taken up in Chapter 6.

Dangers of Bogus Diets

The issue of diet in the treatment of diabetes opens up Pandora's box — a box containing the ill-will deceptions of those seeking profits. This fact is detailed in an article published in U.S. News and World Report, entitled *Diabetes Diet War*.[64] The title's caption states, *"The nutrition advice given to most diabetics might be killing them."*

In this article, called into question was the American Diabetes Association's (ADA) advice for diabetics to eat a high-carbohydrate diet, which is the very thing that leads to diabetes. And, in addition to exacerbating the diabetic condition, high-carbohydrate diets increase the risk of pancreatic cancer in those who already suffer from diabetes.[65] Unfortunately, many doctors, nutritionists, and patients follow this death-dealing advice.

This is the drawback in assuming that a national association's perspective or advice on an issue is correct. What makes it correct? Every position should be challenged and tested. We should not accept any advice on face value.

According to the article, this advice might have been issued to keep people suffering with diabetes from eating high-fat foods, which increase the risk of cardiovascular disease in diabetics. So, instead of cautioning people against eating high-fat foods, the ADA issued a pro-starch dietary format. This does not make sense.

On the other hand, high protein diets pose the risk of renal disease in diabetics. Would-be nutritionists also tout this diet as the best for humans, to the detriment of those who subscribe to this bogus advice.

This article, like many others of its kind, offered no conclusion. It merely served as a battleground for opposing forces to duke it out. This is customary with the mainstream dietary arena. After words are written and spoken, confusion remains, with the diabetes sufferer as the chief casualty.

In preventing and treating diabetes, the assault on the body through overeating must first be stopped. In addition to ceasing gluttony, the type of food consumed must be considered. Consuming large concentrations of carbohydrate-rich foods, particularly cookies, cakes, pies, candies, and processed so-called foods such as macaroni and other plastic-like noodles, increase the risks of diabetes.[66]

Excessive sugar consumption of both natural sugars and artificial sweeteners are linked to the obesity and diabetes pandemics.[67] Researchers have estimated that people living in so-called developed countries consume nearly 250,000 calories of refined sugar each year.[68] This is equivalent to the amount of energy needed to run three marathons a week, year round. Excessive sugar consumption is also linked to many chronic diseases.[69] This is the reason diabetes is a risk factor for other major chronic diseases.

Food biochemical studies have revealed that exposure to both naturally-occurring and man-made toxins have links to diabetes. In the book, *Nuts Are Not Good for Humans: Biological Consequences of Consumption* (by this author), the naturally-occurring toxins that injure the pancreas are detailed. These include protease inhibitors, goitrogens, and several other anti-nutrients. Nuts, as well as other foods, such as beans and certain vegetables, contain these toxins.

Protease inhibitors interfere with the pancreatic digestive enzymes that degrade protein into amino acids for uptake through the intestines. The harm caused by protease inhibitors has long been established. Their inhibitory activity hinders tissue growth and causes pancreatic hypertrophy and hyperplasia, potentially leading to pancreatic cancer.[70]

In this biofeedback system, the pancreas continues to respond to the call for the production of protein-digesting enzymes, thus keeping it continuously working to the detriment of the organ. This unnecessarily burdens the pancreas. Consequently, when the pancreas is stressed and damaged, production of its vital digestive enzymes and hormones (including insulin) is affected. This causes diabetes and other health ailments.

Goitrogens inhibit iodine uptake by the thyroid gland — a major gland that produces hormones that control metabolism. Generally, these hormones affect heart rate, cholesterol level, body weight, energy level, muscle strength, skin condition, menstrual regularity, and memory. These hormones are also important regulators of tissue growth and development, especially in the skeletal, nervous and reproductive systems. Therefore, ingestion of this toxin is linked to obesity and many chronic diseases.

Additionally, thyroid hormones are responsible for carbohydrate metabolism. The hormones stimulate glucose uptake and absorption in cells by working in concert with insulin. Therefore, a reduction in thyroid hormones caused by the goitrogenic inhibition of iodine, leads to a reduction in their interaction with insulin. The result is an increased risk of developing diabetes.

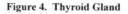

Figure 4. Thyroid Gland

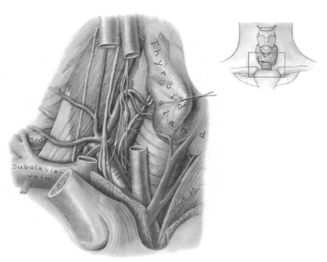

Here we must note that this action might also explain the "insulin-resistance" concept in cells. Because of a low thyroid hormone level, body cells are not able to use insulin as adequately as they require. Thyroid impairment is not atop medical researchers' list of factors that contribute to diabetes.

Unfortunately, many half-learned nutritionists follow the long-held, but incorrect, assumption that nuts and raw vegetables are good for humans to eat. Some researchers have the audacity to recommend nuts as a food to reduce diabetes risks.[71] This, of course, is completely bogus. Most studies that champion nut consumption are absent biochemical studies that show the negative affect of eating protease inhibitors, goitrogens and a host of other natural, but harmful, toxins contained in nuts.

The importance of diet and nutrition in addressing diabetes and other chronic diseases is obvious. Often overlooked, however, is the ingestion of man-made toxins. Most people know that the food supply is contaminated; nevertheless, the adverse health affect of this contamination is not considered in the obesity or diabetes epidemic.

The increased contamination of the environment has kept pace with the rise in chronic disease; therefore, chronic disease prevention and intervention discussions must also include and address the contribution that these poisons lend to the chronic disease epidemic. People must be informed about this contamination and how best to avoid it. This is taken up in the following section and in Chapter 7.

Diabetes-causing Contaminants

Epidemiological data suggest that environmental contamination is associated with diabetes. Of course, we can do little about the toxic atmosphere, and its negative impact on us and on the food we eat. Each breath we take comes with toxins; however, the body mechanisms protect against much of this. We can boost this protection by limiting our exposure to these toxins and allowing the body time to cleanse.

In one study, entitled *Environmental Contaminants as Etiologic Factors for Diabetes*, data showed that the intake of arsenic, nitrates, nitrites, N-nitroso compounds and dioxins such as polychlorinated biphenyls (PCBs) and 2,37,8-tetrachlorodibenzo-p-dioxins (TCDD) increase risk of diabetes.[72] Limiting exposure to these toxins involves proper food selection and preparation. In some cases, the former determines the latter.

For example, the *Nurses' Health Study* showed that consumption of processed meats is positively associated with the risk of type 2 diabetes.[73] This is because nitrites are commonly used for the preservation of meats, and processed meats contain a considerable level of nitrites.

The risk occurs when nitrites combine with the amines in meat. This reaction takes place in either the food or intestine, producing nitrosamines. This toxin has been detected in processed meats, such as sausages and bacon. A word to the wise is sufficient for those who are bent on having their bacon and sausage, along with sand (grits), every morning for breakfast. They are eating themselves into a diabetic condition.

Today, anyone still eating meat is at constant risk of illness and disease, not only from the toxic preservatives, but also through the widespread use of antibiotics, growth promoters, and toxic fertilizers.

Dioxin is the common name used to refer to the chemical, *2,3,7,8-tetrachlorodibenzo-p-dioxin*. Also, other compounds have structures similar to dioxin. These are called dioxin-like compounds or "dioxins", and include:

- Polychlorinated dibenzodioxins (PCDDs);
- Polychlorinated dibenzofurans (PCDFs); and
- Some polychlorinated biphenyls (PCBs)

Dioxins are members of a group of chlorine-based chemicals known as organochlorines. As noted in the name, these chemicals contain chlorine atoms. Chlorine makes the chemicals it binds to more stable against biologic breakdown. Because of this, organochlorines are extremely bioaccumulative and persistent.[74] They accumulate in the food chain and in all mammalian tissues.

Organochlorine insecticides appeared on the market after World War II. They were used in agriculture, and in public health to control insects that transmit diseases, such as mosquitoes. A well-known organochlorine insecticide, *Dichlorodiphenyltrichloroethane* (DDT), was abusively used in farming. Its low-cost made it popular, and farmers overused it. The Honorable Elijah Muhammad warned against the use of DDT in agriculture, and the adverse impact it would have on the population.

In the 1960s, many studies began to report the health risks associated with organochlorines. This eventually caused restrictions to its use in North America and Europe. Albeit, these dangerous chemicals — branded as pesticides, herbicides, fungicides, rodenticides and others — persist in the environment. This contamination is to the extent that the entire atmosphere is poisoned, as these substances are in the very fabric of the earth — soil, air, water, etc.

According to the National Institute of Environmental Health Sciences, dioxin exposure can lead to increased cancer rates, reproductive and developmental problems, increased heart disease, and increased diabetes in humans. The Environmental Protection Agency (EPA) estimates that more than 95% of human exposure to organochlorines, namely dioxins, occurs through food.[75]

A foremost study of dioxins, as a cause of diabetes, is the *Operation Ranch Hand Study*. In this on-going study, researchers are examining the affect of Agent Orange on Vietnam veterans exposed to the herbicide.[76] Agent Orange was used extensively between 1962 and 1971 to destroy the jungle in Vietnam.

The U.S. Air Force began this study because of reports about the adverse health effects occurring in animals exposed to Agent Orange. This study compares the health of 1000 exposed veterans to 1300 Vietnam veterans who did not have contact with Agent Orange.

Although the study is still underway, until 2006, interim results show that veterans exposed to dioxins have a 26% increase in heart disease, with higher levels of circulating dioxin being associated with an increased incidence of hypertension and heart attacks. Additionally, veterans having the highest levels of dioxins in their bodies showed a 47% increase in diabetes.

The study's crafters contend that it still needs to determine if these adverse health effects, essentially diabetes, are independent features of the negative effects of Agent Orange, or something else. What is the *something else*? This is a bogus position, and is in keeping with other government responses to the needs of Vietnam veterans. This response is to "wash over" or hide the truth, and resist providing essential services to remedy the social plight of veterans.

Another epidemiological study, *Linking Dioxins to Diabetes: Epidemiology and Biological Plausibility*, examined the biological mechanisms that might contribute to how dioxins impede glucose transport.[77] The findings revealed the biological workings of how dioxins interfere with the body's natural biofeedback systems.

Another study assessed the relation between exposure to the dioxin, TCDD, and endocrine malfunction. Researchers examined data from the largest morbidity study of industrial workers exposed to TCDD. The findings provided evidence that exposure to TCDD affects thyroid function and glucose metabolism.[78] This study confirmed that obesity and diabetes are, potentially, caused by this type of poison.

Organochlorines are a continuous problem for overweight and obese persons. As previously stated, this fat-soluble chemical compound is stored in adipose tissue. Therefore, accumulation of these compounds in the body is related to body fat mass. Obese and overweight persons have higher organochlorine concentrations than lean persons do.

During weight loss, lipid mobilization and a decrease in fat mass result in increased concentrations of organochlorines in blood plasma and adipose tissue.[79] This means that the risk of adverse health effects from these chemicals also increases.

For example, studies have confirmed adverse relationships between increases in plasma organochlorine concentration and decreases in thyroid hormone (triiodothyronine) concentration; resting metabolic rate, and skeletal muscle markers for fat oxidation. The negative findings have led scientists to recommend strategies that moderately reduce weight, without causing substantial release of organochlorines.[80] This makes sense.

Consider This

We reiterate that the best diet for humans must arise from the goal of longevity. Therefore, it must contain instructions that prevent us from wearing out our digestive organs by ingesting abrasive foods. It must also limit our exposure to natural and synthetic toxins. Finally, it must instruct us on the best foods to eat to obtain adequate nutrition.

Although this world's medical scientists claim that type 2 diabetes is an incurable disease, its pathology indicates that it is, in fact, curable. The person must bring the blood-sugar level back into balance. Medical scientists attempt to do this through pills and potions, to no avail. However, the Honorable Elijah Muhammad writes:[81]

> In regard to you who suffer from sugar diabetes, fasting and staying away from sugar and starchy foods is far better than having your limbs cut off your body because of your foolish carelessness in eating sweets and starchy foods all times of the day…If you have too much sugar in your blood, be careful not to eat any sugar until you get it out.

CHAPTER 4

Causative Factors

Most, if not all, health researchers agree that the cause of obesity includes environmental or societal factors. Generally, these factors comprise the Westernized way of life, the foundational principle of which is to corral wealth and profits. Therefore, every human need has a price tag on it. Food, medicine, education, and the earth's natural resources, such as electricity, water and heating oil are profit centers in this world.

People cannot obtain the necessities of life without money. Just the same, it is through the quest for profit that people are destroyed — as they seek to provide these essentials for themselves and their families. The obesity epidemic is an example of this point — the need for food is being exploited, making people buy and eat more foods and nonfoods than is necessary.

The Scriptures state that the love of money is the root of evil.[82] In the context of this revelation, the Apostle Paul states:

9) But those who desire to be rich fall into temptation and a snare, and into many foolish and harmful lusts, which drown men in destruction and perdition. 10) For the love of money is a root of all kinds of evil, for which some have strayed from the faith in their greediness, and pierced themselves through with many sorrows.

Here, again rests a challenge to those who claim belief in Almighty God. Do we believe this? Is it relevant to the widespread evils of today? What is evil? Evil is that which causes harm, misfortune, or destruction; or anything that impedes the happiness of a person or deprives that person of any good.

According to the Apostle Paul, those desiring riches plunge into foolish and harmful lusts. These demonic persons gain wealth and riches at the expense of other people. These persons are vile bloodsuckers, because they suck the peoples' wealth, while offering nothing of value in return. They sell death; hence, they are *"merchants of death"*.

In acting out their lusts for wealth's sake, they devise and execute evil machinations that ultimately drown people in destruction and perdition. The victims of this gross evil succumb to anguish, misery, suffering, and premature death by means of their money. This is evident in the chronic disease pandemic.

The World Health Organization (WHO) positioned that the burden of chronic diseases is rapidly increasing worldwide.[83] Health experts estimated that, in 2001, chronic diseases contributed approximately 60% of the 56.5 million total reported deaths in the world, and approximately 46% of the global burden of disease. Experts predict that this burden will increase to 57% by 2020.

Considering this assessment, both the obesity and chronic disease pandemics have deprived millions of people of good, especially the greatest good — the gift of life. This means that the root-cause of the obesity epidemic is diabolical, in both intent and implementation. Profit is at the root of this health crisis.

The *merchants of death* use deceit as the primary method to give people destruction in exchange for their wealth. In the healthcare arena, this destruction comes in the form of bogus dietary advice, toxic pills and potions, and brutal surgical procedures. These so-called treatments generate billions of dollars annually. To boot, no healing ever takes place. People die in agony. They die bankrupt of money and of the will to live.

Justifiably, the evildoers do not come away unscathed, with a clean bill of health. As stated by the Apostle Paul, they fall into a snare — *entangled and brought into trouble*. The evildoer's money does not allow him to live in peace and contentment. The evildoer, through his evil schemes, continuously fuels a world that torments his family and him. The evildoer is not in good health, and succumbs to the same diseases as everyone else. The evildoer's lifespan is no longer than the victims. The snare is self-deception, as the evildoer believes that his money separates him from the rest of the human family. It does not.

We need only follow the money to find the root of evil and the evildoers. Let us examine the profit-centered societal factors that cause and promote obesity.

The Terrain

The diet-related chronic disease pandemic, which includes the obesity pandemic, proves that eating is this world's favorite pastime. In addition to eating for nutrition, many people eat to overcome boredom. People eat for entertainment and sport, particularly those who live in the Western world, where food is plentiful.

Eating competitions occur across the world. People travel afar to thrill in these mindless competitions, as they watch to see who can eat the most watermelons, hotdogs, crawl fish, boiled eggs, etc. These people abuse themselves for the sake of bogus titles and foolish honor.

If eating is the most widely engaged sport, then part of the playing field is the food industry. In 2001, Americans spent $738.8 billion on food expenditures, of which $440.4 billion was spent on food prepared at home, and $298.4 billion was spent on food eaten away from home.[84] U.S. food expenditures are projected to rise by 26%, or by $208 billion, between 2000 and 2020.[85]

Thousands of new food products are introduced into the U.S. food market each year. In 1985, approximately 5,500 new food products were introduced. Nearly 10 years later, in 1995, about 17,000 new products were introduced.[86] The total number of food products available in today's marketplace now exceeds 300,000 (although not all at once and not in every store). On average, supermarkets carry 40,000 food items. This compares to the 26,000 items carried ten years ago..[87]

Some health advocates, in their attempt to curb the obesity epidemic, chide the food industry for exacerbating the condition. The following is from an article entitled, *We're Fat and Getting Fatter! What Is the Food Industry's Role?* [88]

> *The (food) industry encourages us to eat by making food easy to obtain; motivates its purchase through taste, convenience, and price; and attempts to bend us to its specific brands through skillful advertising and promotion.*

The article further positions that the battle against obesity and chronic disease is formidable because healthful dietary promotional messages are overcome by the food industry's powerful marketing strategies. For example, in 1997, the food industry was the second largest advertiser in the U.S., with television as the most popular medium.[89] The food industry spent $7 billion on advertising; which was 21 times the $333 million spent by the U.S. Department of Agriculture on nutrition education.

Additionally, the food industry's advertising did not support the national health objectives. We must keep in mind that in a capitalistic society, public and private interests are usually separate and contrary to one another. By public interests, we mean governmental intervention on behalf of its citizenry.

Ironically, the key services in the public's best interests have been gradually put in the hands of private industry. Private or commercial interests now include public health and all that goes with it — medical institutions, healthcare organizations, health insurance organizations, and the pharmaceutical industry, to name a few. This is part of the perils of privatizing governmental responsibilities.

As a profit center, the food industry's objective is to increase sales, and to achieve this, they must promote that which is most appealing and appetizing — sweets and other junk foods. Therefore, the bulk of the food industry's advertising dollars is spent to promote highly processed and packaged junk foods.

Nearly seven times as much money is spent advertising confectionery and snacks, such as candy, gum, mints, cookies, crackers, nuts, chips and other salty snacks, than is spent advertising fruits, vegetables, grains and beans.[89] Such an advertising campaign reveals that children are the primary targets. This is precisely the case.

Health advocates cite that as children enter the elementary and middle school years, societal messages about the role of non-nutritive food become increasingly prevalent and confusing.[90] Rather than addressing the importance of proper nutrition for health, children become targets of advertising for a multitude of unhealthy so-called foods. Children are exposed to an estimated 10,000 advertisements for food per year, 95% of which are for fast foods, candy, sugared cereal and soft drinks.[91]

By the time children reach pre-school, preferences for specific unhealthy foods are already developed.[92] Consequently, encouraging children to break these habits becomes difficult. The blame, however, extends beyond the food industry. Other areas of society lend to the poor dietary habits of children and to the childhood obesity crisis.

For example, millions of American children watch school-based television educational programs that advertise food products including gum, soft drinks, fast food, candy and snack chips.[91] Children are constantly exposed to advertising and vending machines outside the classroom. Meanwhile, nutrition education is infrequent and often inadequate to effectively help children make eating decisions that produce better health.

Overall, the food industry's profiteering quest has produced a similar quest in the health industry, where obesity is now a tremendous profit center.

Obesity Profit Center

The total cost of overweight and obesity is estimated at nearly $130 billion. This is phenomenal. Part of this hefty cost is dispersed as follows:[16]

- $8.8 billion for heart disease related to overweight and obesity;
- $98 billion (in 2001) for type 2 diabetes related to overweight and obesity:[93]
- $21.2 billion for osteoarthritis related to overweight and obesity;
- $4.1 billion for hypertension (high blood pressure) related to overweight and obesity;
- $3.4 billion for gallbladder disease related to overweight and obesity;
- $2.9 billion for breast cancer related to overweight and obesity;
- $933 million for endometrial cancer; and
- $3.5 billion for colon cancer.

These enormous expenditures illustrate the profitability of obesity and suggest that there is an inordinate interest in keeping the population fat. This "interest" also lies in the increased incidence of obesity among children. It means that, in the future, more money must be spent to address this problem.

Clearly, obesity is a cash-cow. This epidemic keeps the nation's profit centers — food, pharmaceuticals, and medical industries — flourishing; and the merchants of death, wealthy. These expenditures go to build and maintain an industry that employs millions of people. Additionally, private investments go into healthcare programs, such as HMOs. This makes disease and early mortality the surest and safest investment opportunities available. There is no doubt that poor health is profitable for many people.

Again, there is also little doubt that those who control the food, health, and scientific industries launch diabolical ploys for profit's sake. Let us consider one such ploy

Diabolical Machinations

In a 1956 report published in Scientific American, entitled *Appetite and Obesity*, a question was posed as to why people overeat and become obese.[42] The author asked: *What factor (or factors) disturbs the mechanism of regulation of food intake in such a way that the balance between intake and energy output is tipped in favor of excessive consumption?* Such a question opened the door to endless scientific studies, because it concerned the biological and biochemical factors associated with overeating. It hypothesized that something natural in the body was being disturbed that caused obesity.

According to the report, scientists conducted research in the 1940s to study the biological mechanisms that control appetite and hunger. Those experiments demonstrated that the central area of the hypothalamus, a segment of the brain, was a "satiety center". Satiety is the state of being satisfactorily full or satisfied. Scientists learned that this part of the brain controlled the hunger or appetite feedback process.

In these studies, researchers destroyed that area of the hypothalamus. As a result, the mice ate profusely, with no regard for satiety. The mice, subsequently, became extremely obese. Some mice weighed 2 to 3 times their normal weight. Comparatively, normal mice, having no brain damage, demonstrated an innate response to their eating habits. For example, after being force-fed until they became obese, the rats refused to eat until they had lost the extra fat accumulated during force-feeding.

Other experiments revealed that brain damage to other areas of the hypothalamus produces the opposite affect — starvation, as the mice had no drive to eat food. Generally, these experiments confirmed that the hypothalamus is the controller of appetite, as well as other biological sensations and drives.

To date, we know that the hypothalamus is an essential part of the autonomic nervous system and has the role of monitoring several body conditions, such as temperature, water balance, metabolism, cardiovascular regulation, and hormone secretion. The hypothalamus also is the center for many drives such as thirst, appetite, and sex. It contains a wide array of neurotransmitters that facilitate and regulate the above functions.

Figure 5. Brain (anterior)

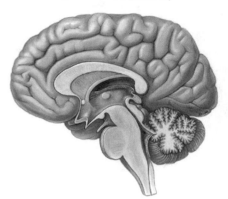

Nearly all neurotransmitters — acetylcholine, noradrenaline, serotonin, dopamine, adrenaline, y-aminobutyric, and glutamate — are contained in the hypothalamus. These substances are vital to brain function. Brain function dictates body function.

The hypothalamus also has a unique relationship with the attached pituitary gland. The pituitary gland is considered the master endocrine gland because it controls the activity of other glands. Its removal or destruction has a tremendous effect on body metabolism, and leads to the atrophy or degeneration of organs, such as the gonads, adrenal, and thyroid glands. The relationship between the hypothalamus and pituitary is very significant, and demonstrates the integration of the nervous and endocrine systems in maintaining homeostasis in the body.

The hypothalamus produces *releasing-hormones*. These hormones regulate the release of other hormones located in the pituitary gland, which affect every part of the human body — by controlling nearly all biological functions. Therefore, anything that injures or negatively affects the hypothalamus disturbs hormonal, behavioral, and autonomic responses.

The *Encyclopedia of Human Biology* describes the detrimental result of damage to the hypothalamus:[94]

> *The importance of these regulatory functions controlled by the hypothalamus cannot be understated. A lesion or deficit in the afferent circuitry, the central organization or the output of the hypothalamus for the control of these homeostatic functions has serious consequences on the individual.*

Hypothalamic injury can cause a number of disorders, including severe organ atrophy, obesity, sleep disturbances, dehydration, and a broad range of emotional imbalances.

Revisiting the obesity study, the researchers concluded:

> *Thinking in terms of first causes, we can trace obesity to three sources: heredity, injury, and unfavorable external factors.*

We briefly addressed the first and third factors — showing that genetics and societal conditions influence overweight and obesity. The second factor, injury, appears obvious because when the brain is injured many body functions are compromised. Some functions are halted, while others are severely modified, causing disease and death.

Interestingly, with respect to this study, scientists injured the brain by using a chemical substance, *gold thioglucose*. As clearly indicated in the name, this is a compound of glucose and gold. This compound caused lesions to the hypothalamus' satiety center.

Gold thioglucose destroyed this area because the glucose dragged the gold into the cells. Scientists purported that the study affirmed that these particular cells, satiety cells, act as sensitive receptors of glucose. This is not surprising because glucose has long been established as the primary energy source of brain cells, as well as all body cells.

Also, not surprising is that the gold was able to permeated the hypothalamus' barrier. Unlike other areas of the brain, the hypothalamus is not a total delimiting brain region. It has a leaky blood-brain barrier because substances, such as hormones and nutrients, must be able to diffuse freely in and out of it.[94]

Perhaps unknown to many is the fact that gold has been used in medicine for centuries.[95] Even at the advent of what is today known as mainstream medicine, studies on the efficacy of gold as a therapeutic remedy were conducted.

For example, the following is recorded in the article, *Gold and Its Relationship to Neurological/Glandular Conditions*:

> *Potter (1894), in his Materia Medica, based on the U.S. Pharmacopoeia of 1890, describes the effects of small doses of gold: "The Salts of Gold promote appetite and digestion…"*

Even then, gold was known to affect appetite. Gold was among the first metals studied for its possible medical affect, preceding the study of most essential elements, such as iron, calcium, etc. Today, the primary therapeutic use of gold is in the treatment of rheumatoid arthritis. Other less common uses include steroid replacement in asthma, treatment of skin disorders, and inclusion in anti-cancer substances.

Shortly after the 1956 gold-thioglucose studies, hundreds of studies were conducted using gold-thioglucose. Brain and endocrine researchers got mileage out of this substance. All studies confirmed the ability of gold-thioglucose as a disrupter of the endocrinological process.

For example, some studies further proved that gold-thioglucose destroys glucose-responsive neurons, validating a previously held hypothesis that glucose-responsive neurons contribute to the long-term regulation of body weight.[96] Another study showed that the biological clock, also called the circadian clock, which is located in the brain, is negatively impacted by destruction of the hypothalamic brain region.[97] Disrupting the body's circadian clock caused disorder of the sleep-wake cycle and other regulated biological systems. These disruptions have profound affects on health.

Fast forwarding to contemporary research, brain-imaging studies in non-human primates has shown that there are sets of neurons in the brain (caudolateral orbitofrontal cortex) that respond to tastes of food only when the animal is hungry.[98] The response of these neurons decreases to nearly zero when the animal has eaten to satiety. When these neurons are destroyed, satiety is not achieved. The animal, therefore, continues to eat and eat — even until death overtakes it.

In light of this, we recognize how difficult it has become to resist eating certain food, especially processed foods that contain artificial chemicals. These adulterated foods sway the appetite, causing greater consumption. Therefore, we must consider that the obesity epidemic might be caused by substances in food — poisons that injure the brain, thereby assassinating the ability of our brains to signal satiety.

Furthermore, foods with a high fat content or high percent of sugar, fat, or a mixture of both, are high in energy density, and promote greater caloric intake. Eating these foods produces an inordinate drive to consume more of these foods. This contributes to food over-consumption.[99] Nutritionists and health officials encourage people to reduce their fat and sugar intake, although this is challenging to do. People are prone to eat foods they enjoy, and these high energy-dense foods are the more tasteful foods. They are also the most adulterated foods.

The enormous consumption of sugar is connected to the country's health problems. There are hundreds of additives used in foods, and more are being approved each year.[100] Artificial sweeteners are among several major categories of food additives, and are found in most foods. So, it is not difficult to conceive that the onslaught of obesity may be the result of the diabolical and premeditated act to adversely affect the hypothalamus.

We should not be so arrogant or naïve to think that food adulteration is not also used for the express purpose of disturbing the natural biological workings of the brain and digestive systems. Unfortunately, too many people shun the thought of "conspiracy", much less sound evidence that confirms high-level and broad-based conspiracies. They are quick to reply, "I am not interested in your conspiracy theories."

Yet, does not a person need to conspire to get another person to undergo or succumb to that, which is unnatural and destructive? Would not something natural be as unassuming as flowing water? In this case, good health is something that most people overlook when they have it, because good health does not disturb anyone.

On the other hand, bad health — sickness and disease — is one of the most disturbing things to confront. To conspire means *to plan together secretly to commit an illegal or wrongful act or accomplish a legal purpose through illegal action*. With gross illegal dealings, anguish, sorrow, death, and destruction all around us, it seems that plenty of conspiring has been going on and is underway.

The disease pandemic, therefore, must be the result of deliberate and premeditated machinations.

Additionally, when it comes to obesity, why is it easier to gain weight than ever before; hence, the obesity and super obesity pandemics? Why does such a condition correspond with the ever-increasing introduction and marketing of chemical-sprayed natural foods, chemical-laden processed foods, and chemical-injected meats? Do these things have anything to do with obesity? Of course, they do.

In the past decade, scientists have uncovered much more about the biological regulation of appetite, particularly that its regulation is chemically-coded in the hypothalamus.[101] Any derangement in this signaling network produces an excessive drive for food.

Figure 6. Brain

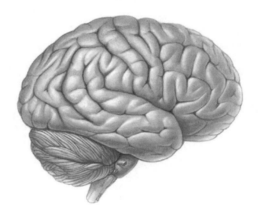

Scientists have identified and characterized a multitude of neurotransmitters and other neuro-factors that promote, transmit, or terminate the electrical impulses that drive appetite. The weight-controlling biological substances are located in both the brain and adipose tissue.[37]

Moreover, scientists have identified the precise pathways containing these signaling molecules, and the intricate interconnections among them. The following summarizes the major aspects of appetite regulation. [101]

1. Embedded in the networks controlling a multitude of
   hypothalamic functions, there is a distinct circuitry regulating

appetite. This circuitry is composed of an interconnected network of pathways elaborating and emitting orexigenic and anorexigenic signals...

2. The neurons producing these orexigenic and anorexigenic signal molecules are subject to modulation by the internal milieu comprised of a variety of hormonal and other biologically active molecules...

3. A cascade of temporally related neural events in various components of the appetite-regulating network (ARN) precedes feeding episodes.

4. Emerging evidence supports the involvement of a distinct neural device for the timely onset of appetite expression, and disintegration of this control may result in unregulated food consumption.

5. A deficit in availability of orexigenic signals at the signal transduction level, whether temporary or permanent, can perturb the postsynaptic receptor dynamics that eventuate in hyperphagia and increased body weight gain indistinguishable from that produced by excessive production and release of orexigenic signals.

6. Co-existence and co-release of orexigenic signals, along with the redundant overlapping and interconnected orexigenic and anorexigenic signaling pathways within the hypothalamus, provide a microenvironment wherein subtle perturbations shift signaling in favor of unregulated hyperphagia rather than anorexia.

There is much in these findings, which can be used to aid the population into better health or to destroy the population for greed's sake. For example, among the "good" in these findings is the importance of regulating one's diet. When our diets are unregulated, we create an environment where our body constantly signals for food, despite the fact that it does not need it.

Generally, the *bad* is the obesity and chronic disease pandemics. More specifically, we draw the conclusion that this scientific knowledge was and is used for evil purposes from the following facts.:

• Also, the use of chemical additives in food, especially artificial sweeteners and dyes, is pervasive throughout the food supply.

- The rise in obesity is commensurate with the advancement in the knowledge of neuronal regulation of appetite;
- Obesity is a profit-center, and is the leading adverse health condition driving healthcare costs into the trillions of dollars; and
- The food industry's growth and profits are inordinate.

The process of drug development sheds some light on how these biological findings could be easily manipulated through chemicals added to our food. For example, diabetes researchers, through experiments with the adipocyte cell, purport that an antidiabetic drug could be developed that interfere with the inner workings of the cells.[102]

We should not be dismayed in learning, one day, that the *merchants of death* have used chemicals to upset the natural workings of the human body. Many people already know that this is exactly the case, right now. This is sheer evil.

Food Additives

On that last point, let us take up the controversy surrounding the use of food chemicals. Today, man-made or synthetic food chemicals are ubiquitous throughout the food chain — that is, on the food and in the food; in the manufacturing process; and in the packaging materials that contain the foods.

The Food and Drug Administration (FDA) regulates food additives. According to the FDA, additives are necessary because they help keep food *wholesome and appealing while en route to markets sometimes thousands of miles away from where it is grown or manufactured*.[102] The FDA states that additives also improve the nutritional value of certain foods and can make them more appealing by improving their taste, texture, consistency and color.

The Agency also notes that food additives can be used to adulterate the food by making bad or spoiled foods appear safe and wholesome to eat. It cautions food handlers not to engage these unscrupulous tactics.

However, we know that many manufacturers adulterate foods. The FDA or the USDA cannot effectively monitor the dealings throughout the food industry. This means that we should realize the food supply is not totally safe.

The following table lists the FDA's food additive categories.

Table 4: Food Additives Categories

• Anticaking agent	• Hormone
• Antifoaming (or defoaming) agent	• Inhibitor
• Antioxidant	• Miscellaneous
• Boiler compound	• Natural substances and extractives
• Bleaching agent or flour-maturing agent	• Non-nutritive sweetener
• Buffer and neutralizing agent	• Nutrient
• Component or coating for fruits & vegetables	• Nutritive Sweetener
• Dietary supplement	• Pesticide other than fumigant
• Emulsifier	• Chemical preservative
• Enzyme	• Sanitizing agent for food processing equipment
• Essential oil and/or oleoresin (solvent free)	• Solubilizing and dispersing agent
• Substances under the Food Additives Amendment added directly to feed	• Sequestrant
• Natural flavoring agent	• Solvent
• Substance used in conjunction with flavors	• Spices, other natural seasonings & flavorings
• Fumigant	• Spray adjuvant
• Fungicide	• Stabilizer
• Herbicide	• Synthetic flavor

Some food additives are also addictive. Among the well-known cases of how adulterated foods cause addiction was brought to light in the French fries debacle. Addictive agents were added to fast food products.[103] These chemicals affect the neurological workings that control satiety and appetite, demonstrating the diabolical intent of food manufacturers. Again, this practice is directly linked to obesity and chronic diseases.

FDA officials state that some additives could be eliminated if people were willing to grow their own food, harvest and grind it, spend many hours cooking and canning, or accept increased risks of food spoilage. Before the industrial age, these were the very things people did. Foods were harvested locally, and no one complained about having to do it.

The *merchants of death* have connived to de-localize agriculture and food distribution, creating mega agribusinesses — which is dependent on man-made chemicals. Again, as stated by the Apostle Paul, greed is the cause of this widespread evil, in the name of convenience, science and medicine.

CHAPTER 5

This World's Treatment

The deliberate obscurity placed on the cause of obesity has created financial opportunities for government institutions, medical, food and pharmaceutical industries, as well as varying forms of quackery. These financial opportunities are so colossal that obesity, alone, should be considered an industry. Again, this environment is the same today as it was centuries ago. The dietary dark ages persist.

Many medical scientists agree that weight loss improves the adverse health consequences associated with obesity, including high blood pressure, diabetes, and elevated blood-lipid levels.[105] Weight loss as small as 5% to 10% has been shown to benefit a person's health. This appears very logical — for if increased weight brings about disease, then reduced weight should alleviate those conditions.

Weight loss, therefore, has become the primary objective for eliminating obesity and its related health disorders. Obesity treatments focus on weight loss. Here, we must reinforce the fact that weight loss, as a primary objective, falls short of the overall goal of health. Longevity is the overall goal of health. Because such a goal cannot be achieved when a person is overweight, weight loss is inherent in the solution, but it should not be the chief focus.

As previously noted throughout this book, the central and most controversial issue involves the particular treatments used to reduce a person's weight. The manner in which weight is reduced can injure the person by traumatizing the body. This can lead to severe health problems, including death.[35] History is filled with examples of this.

In this world's treatment, the primary therapies used to treat obesity are dietary, pharmaceutical, and surgical. Some of these treatments, particularly drugs and dietary advice, make their way into the marketplace through clinical studies. Federal, state, and local government sometimes sponsor and support this research. This is their way of protecting the public from bogus, unproven treatments that claim to solve obesity.

Some of this research is also supported and funded by private companies. These companies usually have a vested interest in the disease. For example, pharmaceutical companies often sponsor and facilitate clinical trials to test the effectiveness of drugs developed for treating diseases. Given this, there is always the chance that the research is tainted or bias for profit's sake.

Many clinical trials for obesity are underway. Many have already been completed. These include trials for various drugs, nutrients, and dietary and exercise regimens. For example, exercise-related trials include those that assess strength training following gastric bypass surgery;[106] or exercise training in so-called "obesity-prone" Black and Caucasian women.[107]

Nutrient-related trials include the testing of substances hypothesized to reduce obesity or reduce obesity-related risk factors. For example, *Quercetin*, a so-called natural compound that allegedly slows carbohydrate digestion, is being tested as a component that can be placed in foods to help diabetics.[108]

Obesity drug-related clinical trials test drugs that fall in the following classes: anorectics, beta3-adrenoceptor agonists, central stimulants, hormones, lipase inhibitors and serotonin uptake inhibitors.

The outcomes of these trials determine whether the drug or substance is approved and marketed to the consumer. The design of the trial or study is at the heart of the decision to either approve or reject the drug or substance. This is the most controversial aspect of clinical trials because the designs some studies assure outcomes favorable to the drug or substance in question. This is very common today. In many cases, studies become advertisements, not only to approve the substance, but also to influence consumers to purchase them.

Diet Controversies

By now, most of us are aware that many dietary plans and programs exist. There are as many diet plans as there are people who want to become self-appointed nutritionists. This means that scores of diet plans and programs exist, as too many people believe they know the best way to eat. In fact, the rate of obesity runs neck-to-neck with the number of people dieting. Surveys reveal that most adults are trying to lose weight or maintain normal weight.[109] Some recent figures show that approximately 54 million Americans are dieting.[110]

In the past 20 years, alone, we have learned of diets that advise people to eat anything, and to eat at anytime, even continuously. Some diets promote the consumption of fats. Some feature starches. Others tout protein. Yet, others advise consumption of all these, in hefty amounts.

Some people are advised to eat raw foods only — vegetables, grass, beans, leaves, etc. They call themselves "raw foodists". Other people are advised to eat only cooked foods. Still others are told to eat no food, but instead to drink "power" shakes and vegetable juices. Then, there are those who claim to get everything they need from the air, having no need for food.

Of course, much of this is ridiculous and false, and goes against the law of life. This is the reason death runs rampant despite the millions of dietary books currently available on the market. The prevalence of overweight and obesity continues to increase.

Evidence shows that many dieters succeed in taking weight off, but very few, approximately 5% to 10%, are successful at keeping the weight off over the long-term.[111] This is primarily because many highly-touted diets fail to address the purpose of food. In addition, the aim of too many authors of diet books is to make a buck.

If there is something good about the obesity epidemic, it is its formidability against bogus diets. It brings everyone face-to-face with the efficacy of his or her lifestyle and dietary regimen. In other words, no lightweight, unscientific diet program is successful. Obesity continues to steamroll over the plentiful, substandard and inept dietary advice and recommendations, even from the government.

Government-sanctioned Advice

For example, the *Dietary Guidelines for Americans*, developed jointly by the Departments of Health and Human Services (HHS) and Agriculture (USDA), are issued to provide recommendations to Americans about proper diet and nutrition. These recommendations are supposedly based on current scientific knowledge of food, diet and nutrition. Additionally, the Guidelines form the basis of Federal food, nutrition education, and information programs.

The Guidelines were initially published in 1980, then revised and reissued every five years — 1985, 1990, 1995 and 2000.[112] Although the advice has been modified each issue, the common denominator among them is the promotion to eat many, many meals. These Guidelines contain no meal-time frequency parameters, meaning how often a person should eat (that is, 1, 2, or 3 meals a day). Therefore, those who follow it will find themselves eating too much and too often. People will find themselves obese.

To further exacerbate this futile guidance, the government has issued other dietary programs that do the same — promote gluttony. The latest is the *5 A Day for Better Health Program*.[113] This is the nation's largest public-private nutrition education initiative with so-called *5 A Day* coordinators in each state or territory, championing this form of gluttony. Foolishly, the Program's goal is to increase fruit and vegetable consumption of every American to five servings a day by 2010. This simply means eating five meals a day.

Again, does not these government-sanctioned dietary programs mirror the same advice delivered in the 18th and 19th centuries, which made overeating a national habit? Is not this advice a contributor to the long-standing obesity epidemic? How will eating five meals a day curtail the obesity crisis? It will not! It will only make it worst.

Sadly, this advice is being heavily promoted in the Black community — a community already burdened by obesity and obesity-related chronic diseases. Uninformed Black radio and television personalities are pushing this false and deadly guidance, to the detriment of their own people. They are working in cooperation with health agencies to push unproven, death-dealing programs on the people, while believing that they are doing the best thing. They are ignorant and unaware of the ploys of the *merchants of death*.

However, I do understand their position. Yes, this dietary advice is government-stamped, which should make it true. Yes, this dietary advice seems logical, as eating fruits and vegetables are natural, healthy foods. Nevertheless, this advice is dangerous, and follows the same pattern as other government-sanctioned advice. Additionally, this advice will produce the same results — worsen the health crisis.

No government-sanctioned dietary advice has improved health. In fact, no mainstream dietary advice has improved the health of the populations. Both sources hurl long-held dietary assumptions and fallacies.

Known Fallacies

Among many dietary fallacies is the long-held position that eating dietary fat causes obesity. Nutritionists, after recognizing that elevated blood-lipid levels played a role in obesity and chronic disease, blamed dietary fat for all of this.[114] They believed that a reduction in the fat intake would lead to a 'spontaneous' reduction in body weight and better health.[115]

In attempting to prove this position, researchers conducted many studies, most of which were bogus. Nonetheless, it appeared that they did prove their point. Food manufacturers responded with a slew of adulterated food products.

This led to the low-fat, fat-free, and reduced-fat food explosion. Every food had a fat-free counterpart for those wanting the same foods, but with less fat in them. People spent billions of dollars on these adulterated, chemical-concocted processed foods. As we know, these monetary and dietary efforts did not curtail the obesity or chronic disease epidemics. Matters got worse.

This was because people felt free to eat low-fat and fat-reduced foods. They were deceived, as they believed that replacing the 3 or 4 fat-laden meals they ate each day with the 3 or 4 fat-reduced meals would lead to weight loss and better health. Again, no meal-time frequency or food intake parameters were given to them. People just ate, and ate, and ate.

It was realized that not only was dietary fat converted to fat and stored in adipose tissue, but also excess proteins and carbohydrates traveled the same course. People were not aware of this — that other elements in the food were converted into fat and added to their storehouse of fat. Scientific researchers knew this, as this is basic physiology, but it was not conveyed as intensely as it should have been. This reaffirms the fact that every human being should be armed with knowledge of human physiology and anatomy.

Another dietary moneymaking plot that came on the heels of the low-fat/reduced fat debacle was the reduced-energy nonsense. Studies began to appear that supported the hypothesis that it was not *reduced-fat*, but the reduction of the total energy in foods that produces weight loss. Consequently, food manufacturers responded with reduced-calorie foods. These also flooded the market. And, people do the same with these as they do with the reduced-fat foods — eat them all day and all night. The result is also the same. People are getting fatter.

So again, a gullible population, looking for a quick fix to a metabolic problem fell for another trick. Actually, they continue to fall for tricks, as both types of adulterated foods are still pervasive throughout the market.

Largely, this entire fiasco can be blamed on so-called health researchers and their slanted scientific research. They engage short-term studies, and offer the results of these studies as proof that they proved their hypotheses. Short-term studies are experiments that last under a year. Studies on the long-term efficacy of dietary programs have been few and far between.[116] The reason is that long-term studies reveal less success.

To date, it is quite evident that short-term dietary studies in obese persons intrinsically show noticeable changes. These short-term studies show modest and noteworthy reductions in body weight.[117] However, if consumption habits remain the same, despite the change in food items, people gradually regain the weight, as their bodies adapt to storing a new type of food to the fat depots.

Any sudden change in one's diet will register an immediate change. Short-term studies run the breath of these sudden changes. On the other hand, long-term studies revealed compensatory mechanisms that eradicated any weight loss experienced in the "newness" stage of the dietary regimen. This was so even in diets that featured only modest consumption of dietary fat — within the range of 18% - 40% of total energy.

One assessment of the efficacy of low-fat diets concluded:[118]

Diets high in fat are not the primary cause of the high prevalence of excess body fat in our society, and the failure of a reduction in the percentage of energy from fat to reduce obesity in Western populations is consistent with the results of long-term randomized trials.

This also holds true for reduced-energy diets. Also true is that none of these "reduced" dietary regimens are without cases of injury to the dieter. For example, in 1978, 17 deaths were reported from very-low-calorie diets containing collagen as the principal source of protein.[119] People are injured daily by following the multitudes of dietary plans. This is especially so with imbalance diets that focus on large intakes of specific nutrients, and reductions in or elimination of other nutrients in one's diet.

The *merchants of death* keep people entangled in foolish dietary quests by pointing them to *this* or *that* food, or to *this* or *that* dietary plan. Meanwhile, the most essential factor is omitted or purposely hidden. This factor is eliminating gluttony. Research that substantiates how often an adult should eat has been avoided, so people never consider that they should not eat as often as they do.

For example, should we, as adults, continue to eat the same number of meals we ate when we were babies or toddlers — 2 to 4 meals a day? During those years, we were still growing, so food for growth was necessary. Is the amount of food required for growth the same as that required for maintenance, after growth has stopped? Are we still justified in eating 3, 4 or 5 meals a day?

We must reconcile the apparent logic, which is, how can obesity or chronic disease be alleviated without diets that include food consumption or intake parameters? This issue is taken up in Chapter 6.

Obesity Drugs

The current explosion in genetic research, combined with the drive of pharmaceutical companies to discover effective anti-obesity pills and potions, has directed obesity remedies toward treatment rather than prevention.[120] Although, some drug companies attempt to paint their nostrums as prevention efforts, this is not the case.

When considering obesity and diabetes drugs, we must keep several facts in mind. First, and to reiterate, today's prescription drug industry is an outgrowth of the quackery debacle of the 18th and 19th centuries, which featured bogus nostrums, such as *Daffey's Elixir Salutis, Bateman's Pectoral Drops*, and *Hooper's Female Pills*. Many other nostrums flooded the marketplace, and commanded the public's dollar by promising magical and mystical cures.

People were not cured after ingesting most of these potions. They also were injured, as some of these so-called remedies contained highly toxic chemicals. As we have stated, little has changed. There is enough history to support this fact. Most of us can attest to having been injured after ingesting a pill or potion.

Today's pharmaceutical industry generates approximately $130 billion annually.[121] The nutraceutical industry gathers another $17 billion from the American consumer.[122] Nutraceuticals are food and drinks that promise some medical benefit, and includes products such as vitamins, protein and energy bars and drinks, and a host of other so-called health-promoting concoctions. This market is expected to grow by leaps and bounds, as people attempt to prevent and treat diseases themselves.

Figure 7. Money for Pills

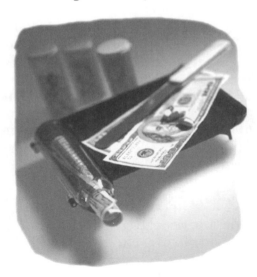

The second point is a reminder of the root of disease. This root is injurious lifestyle behaviors with particular emphasis on improper diet. In the books, *How To Eat To Live*, the Honorable Elijah Muhammad states that the commercialization of food has put divinely forbidden and poison foods on the market, and that consuming these so-called foods is causing the epidemics of disease and early death. The nostrum industry is an outgrowth of this travesty. The pharmaceutical industry develops and markets chemicals to counteract the poisons in the food.

The tremendous growth of pharmaceutical sales over the past few decades supports this position. In the U.S. General Accounting Office's financial assessment of pharmaceutical expenditures, several factors contributing to the wide use of prescription drugs in America were identified.[123] One factor was the ever-increasing chronic disease epidemic.

For example, the number of U.S. citizens with arthritis increased from an estimated 38 million in 1990 to 70 million in recent years. This equates to one-third of the U.S. adult population having the disease. And, as previously noted, obesity and diabetes have steadily increased, causing other associated diseases to increase, as well. The effort to treat these conditions has produced significant sales for the pharmaceutical industry.

Finally, obesity drugs are not on record as having cured anyone of any disease.[124] Of late, the contrary, injury, has been the experience for many people.[4] This is partly due to the greed of drug companies to concoct a "blockbuster" drug as an effort to make substantial profits. However, the failure of drugs to heal and cure is not new. Nor is the injurious failure of obesity drugs new.

For example, *thyroid extract*, first used during the late 1800s, was a promised remedy for treating obesity.[125] The result was an overactive thyroid gland that produced hyperthyroidism, a life-threatening condition with catabolic consequence to bones, muscles, and the heart. Those taking this potion gradually fell to pieces.

Later, the drug, *dinitrophenol*, was used in the 1930s. Among the many reactions users experienced, neuropathy and cataracts were most notable. Neuropathy is a disease or abnormality of the nervous system. The cataracts caused impaired vision and blindness. These adverse affects led to the discontinuance of this deadly nostrum.[126]

This disaster was followed by the introduction of amphetamine in 1937.[127] Reports of addiction soon followed. This drug, although manipulating the neuronal network to produce weight loss, also caused mental disorders. Thereafter, chemicals structurally similar to amphetamine were branded as addictive agents or "get high" drugs. This still did not curtail their use in obesity treatments. People were willing to surrender their mental stability to lose a few pounds. Unfortunately, many people still think this way.

Decades following, anorexigenic drugs, such as amphetamines, digitalis, and diuretics, caused an epidemic of primary pulmonary hypertension. This condition caused vast injury and death. The deadly result led to public hearings by the U. S. Senate. This, of course, meant nothing — except future votes for those politicians who took up the issue in response to public outcry.

This was not the case in Europe. In 1971, the appetite suppressant, *aminorex* or *aminoxaphen*, was taken off the market in Europe after an outbreak of pulmonary hypertension was linked to its use.[128] The U.S. did not follow suit.

Research revealed that appetite suppressants were not only associated with primary pulmonary hypertension, but also caused inhibition of voltage-gated potassium channels, membrane depolarization, and calcium entry in pulmonary artery smooth muscle cells.[129] This means that the adverse health affects of appetite suppressants operate at the molecular level, altering vital processes. The drugs damage the cells and discombobulate critical body systems. It also means that a hosts of other ailments, which have not been acutely identified, also pound the users of these drugs.

In rebellion against that which is sensible, the U.S. has experienced a most recent disaster with appetite suppressant drugs — the phen-fen and Redux tragedy.[130] Redux was the first obesity drug approved by the FDA in 25 years. It was approved in April 1996. After ringing up a toll of death and bodily destruction for more than a year, the FDA banned it from the market. This occurred in September 1997.

The drug was linked to deaths and injuries from serious coronary and pulmonary conditions. Symptoms associated with the drug included chest pains, shortness of breath, and rapid or irregular heartbeat. However, most overlooked was the brain damage it caused. People became insane.

This ban came as two other obesity drugs, Orlistat and Sibutramine, were in the approval pipeline. The ban of Redux sent shock waves through the pharmaceutical industry, affecting the two other drugs. The manufacturer of Orlistat, temporarily withdrew its drug application. Additionally, the manufacturer of Sibutramine, which had received a letter of approval from the FDA and had originally planned to market the drug in late-1997, delayed its launch. Perhaps both companies were laying low until the Redux storm subsided. Today, these two nostrums are the leading obesity drugs currently on the market.

In the first edition of *Obesity, Diabetes, & How To Eat To Live*, which was published before the ban of Redux, I dedicated an entire chapter to the FDA's diabolical and politically-motivated approval of this deadly drug. This chapter is in Appendix A. The evil machinations involved in approving this drug points to the need of citizen involvement in drug reviews. At the very least, this bogus process should be absent commercial influence. Let us continue.

The Redux crash made pharmaceutical companies skeptic about pursuing the obesity market. According to some health researchers, the poor safety and efficacy track-records of previous obesity drugs were among several factors that stymied aggressive investment by pharmaceutical companies in obesity drug development.[131] Another factor was indifference and ignorance by the medical profession, who often were careless in prescribing the drugs. Their negligence was too great of a risk factor for drug companies.

Another factor was the lack of molecular targets for drug discovery. An obesity gene was needed. None has been found, but the search continues.

The resurgence of obesity drug discovery is linked to the alleged advances in molecular biology, as it pertains to understanding the mechanisms that drive normal energy homeostasis and obesity. We can rest assure that the forecasted $200 billion obesity market was the main driving force behind this resurgence.[1]

Additionally, 5 to 10 years might be long enough for people to forget the phen-fen/Redux tragedy, making a new breed of obesity drugs potentially more successful. The problem/failed-solution recycling process is underway.

Admittedly, drug developers know that developing new obesity drugs is a tall order. Researchers record:[1]

> *...from a scientific and commercial perspective, this area of drug development is fraught with difficulty and uncertainty. Orlistat, for example, is the biggest selling anti-obesity drug (worldwide sales of $600 million in 2001), but unpleasant side-effects and modest weight loss have compromised the clinical and commercial success of the product, especially in non-North American countries.*

Sibutramine, a mixed serotonin-noradrenaline reuptake blocker, has encountered similar difficulties (lower-than-expected sales of $200 million in 2001) due mainly to cardiovascular side-effects and a cool reception from regulatory authorities.

We must note that Sibutramine has proved most potent in disrupting pulmonary arteries.[129] Yet, it is still on the market in America. Meanwhile, Europe has banned appetite suppressant drugs.[132] Europe has a vigilant population, who are always ready to battle the greedy *merchants of death*, especially those in the U.S., who seek to spread their death-dealing products to other countries.

Current obesity drugs, as well as those in the pipeline, are classified according to several categories. These are:

- *Centrally-acting appetite suppressants*, which work primarily by increasing the availability of anorexigenic neurotransmitters (noradrenaline, serotonin and dopamine).
- *Peripherally-acting* drugs that enhance energy expenditure, slow gastric emptying and create a heightened sense of fullness, or inhibit fat absorption.
- *Compounds* already licensed to treat other health conditions. For example, the atypical antidepressant, bupropion, which is licensed for smoking cessation, may also reduce body weight. Similarly, topiramate, a novel anti-epileptic agent, has favorable effects in some obese subgroups.

In the most recent study of a "probable obesity potion", scientists noting that the gut hormone fragment peptide YY_{3-36} (PYY), reduces appetite and food intake when infused into subjects of normal weight, ventured to examine the presence of this hormone in people suffering from obesity.[133] They concluded that obese persons were not resistant to the anorectic effects of PYY, but had low levels of this hormone, which they implored may contribute to the pathogenesis of obesity.

The verdict of this research is that a pill that contains this hormone might reduce obesity. This is absolutely ridiculous, yet this might be the next obesity wonder drug. We should not wonder if it will work. It will not!

Diabetes Drugs

Diabetes drugs have not been left out of this grotesque picture. Rezulin (troglitazone), a highly touted diabetes drug, was marketed in 1997 after the FDA's approval. Shortly thereafter, the FDA began issuing warnings linking the drug to liver damage. The FDA called this damage side-affects despite the fact that permanent injury and deaths were resulting. How is something that causes death a side-effect? Again, the play with words causes many people to miss the logic.

While these warnings caused Great Britain to ban the drug, the U.S. government continued to market it. In fact, the FDA resisted banning the drug in a most notorious and arrogant fashion. Approximately 40 cases of acute liver failure — most of them resulting in death, and some requiring liver transplants — caused a public uproar. It was a replay of the Redux scandal. Consumer groups called for the withdrawal of the drug, but the FDA responded by convening a panel.

This panel, the Endocrinologic and Metabolic Drugs Advisory Committee, recommended continued use of the drug, to the delight of the drug's manufacturer, Parke-Davis/Warner-Lambert. The Panel issued bogus recommendations to show that it had considered the dangers of the drug. These included requiring *increased patient education, frequent liver monitoring* for those taking the drug, and *new labeling* detailing usage recommendations. This was a sham in the truest sense of the word.

The Panel insisted that the benefits Rezulin provided outweighed its detriments. How is it that a drug that kills, instead of helps, has a benefit? The gift of life is the greatest benefit. Therefore, the loss of it due to toxic pills is unacceptable. However, because the "dollar" is valued above all, a person's life is expendable, with no associated remorse. People are no more than test animals in the face of big business.

Fortunately, the persistence of consumer groups and the growing fears surrounding the continued use of the drug forced the FDA to surrender to reason, logic, and intelligence — traits that are absent the political climate of big business. The ban came as the death toll, allegedly, reached 63, accompanying 90 confirmed cases of liver failure. Most likely, more people suffered, than was reported, especially when nearly a million people used the drug. Lawsuits continue to fly. Rezulin, however, had generated nearly $2 billion in sales before it was banned. Does the deadly nostrum, *Radithor,* come to mind?

There are more than a dozen diabetes drugs on the market, each one promising relief, while posing imminent danger to the consumer. Appendix B contains the current list of these death-dealing drugs and the dangers they pose. At least, anyone already taking these drugs and those considering taking them will know what to expect. Again, the manufacturers call these biological reactions to these drugs *side-effects* when they are risk factors. All diabetes drugs cause adverse reactions to critical biofeedback systems.

For example, nearly all diabetes drugs pose the risk of causing low-blood sugar levels. Therefore, consumers must expect to contend with the conditions that result from this. For example, symptoms of *mild low blood-sugar* may include blurred vision, cold sweats, dizziness, fast heartbeat, fatigue, headache, hunger, light-headedness, nausea, and nervousness. Symptoms of more *severe low blood-sugar* may include disorientation, pale skin, seizures, shallow breathing, and ultimately, coma, leading to death.

Additionally, contraindications are associated with every drug, including diabetes and obesity drugs. A contraindication is a factor that renders the administration of a drug inadvisable. In layman's terms, these are health preconditions. For example, diabetic ketoacidosis, inflammatory bowel disease, colonic ulceration or partial intestinal obstruction are preconditions that eliminate many diabetes drugs as treatment options.

We must mention that many decades ago, the Honorable Elijah Muhammad warned those suffering from diabetes not to use drugs to control their blood-sugar level. People are steadily learning why they should not use drugs. To their detriment, the lessons are hard-learned.

Drugs: What Are They

It is evident that many, if not most, people have not really thought about what is contained in the pills they are swallowing. Perhaps they do not quite see those pills as chemicals. Nevertheless, this is exactly what they are. The July 7, 1995 issue of

Chemical & Engineering News published an article entitled, *Fine And Intermediate Chemicals Makers Emphasize New Products and Processes*. The caption read, *Rise in competition and pressures on cost, especially in the pharmaceutical sector, force technological innovations*. The article reads:

> *Of the $42 billion of fine chemicals sold annually worldwide, the drug industry uses $12.6 billion worth, or 30% of the total. True, the pesticide industry's $14.7 billion, 35% share is greater.*

To date, sales of fine chemicals are over $52 billion.[134] Fine chemicals are pure, single substances that are produced by specific chemical reactions. They are bought and sold based on their chemical identity. Pharmaceutical fine chemicals include both intermediates for drug production and bulk active drugs. These chemicals are compounded with inert pigments, solvents, and fillers — called excipients — and made into dosage forms.

Figure 2 shows how *fine* chemicals are used. Bulk medicinals comprise 30% of fine chemical use, while pesticides use a bit more, 35%. These chemicals, therefore, are used in agriculture and medicine. They also comprise the artificial flavors in foods and drinks — for example, producing the tastes of strawberries and oranges without either fruit being in the food or drink.

What does this mean? It means that we have popped, in pill form, the same chemicals we just ate in the food. So, if the chemicals in the food caused the illness or disease, then how can these same chemicals, now in pill form, solve the illnesses? Realistically, they cannot and they do not.

Figure 8. "Fine" chemical sales distribution

Distribution of "fine" chemicals

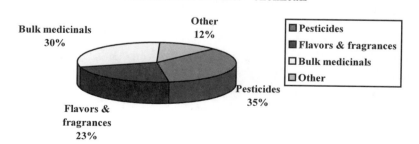

Bulk medicinals 30%

Other 12%

Flavors & fragrances 23%

Pesticides 35%

- Pesticides
- Flavors & fragrances
- Bulk medicinals
- Other

In addition, some people may be wearing these same chemicals in the high-priced perfume, with the fancy Italian name, they spray on their cheeks and neck. These same chemicals makeup the perfume and cologne we wear. According to the chart, this use represents 23% of fine chemical sales.

One would think that if these chemicals had any healing powers, then we should be healed, indeed, especially after eating them through the food and drugs, and wearing them on our bodies. The *merchants of death* are laughing at us, as they count our money.

This is not to suggest that there are no benefits in drugs. Drugs temporarily relieve the discomfort of the ailment. A greater concentration of chemicals contained in a pill can overpower other, less dense, chemicals in our bodies. This does not mean that the biological cell is in good shape. It only means that the *concentrated* chemicals are winning the battle against the toxins already in our bodies. We should not make our bodies constant and continuous arenas for the "battle of the toxins". As we have learned, these arenas will not last very long under chemical skirmishes.

Drug Interactions

Here, we must also note additional dangers incurred with the use of drugs. The unprecedented prescription drug use in the U.S. has brought concerns regarding *drug-to-drug* and *drug-to-food* interactions.

Why is there such a thing as an adverse food-to-drug or drug-to-drug interaction? The human body has a host of activity taking place within it. This activity is what makes us live. It involves the constant replenishing, rejuvenation, and regeneration of the body. Overall, numerous biochemical processes occur, and when new substances — whether food or drugs — enter the body through ingestion, more chemical reactions result. Some of these reactions are beneficial, while others are not. When these reactions are adverse, human life is threatened.

According to the U.S. General Accounting Office, prescribing errors and drug mishaps cost more than $20 billion per year.[135] Many people have been severely injured or killed from these mishaps. One report states that over two million people are hospitalized each year and as many as 140,000 people are killed from the side-effects related to various prescription drugs.[136]

As astounding as this might appear, we have witnessed adverse chemical reactions in our daily living. For example, how many of us have mixed ammonia with bleach or with another potent cleanser? This chemical reaction produces extremely pungent and intolerable fumes, which literally drives the person out of the room.

The thought of drinking the mixture does not even enter the mind, because the fumes are enough of an attack. Inhaling these fumes can cause serious injury, even death. Any doubt that these two chemicals do not mix well is eliminated. In fact, this is how liquid explosives are made — two or more chemicals combine to produce a deadly reaction.

According to an investigative report in the U.S. News and World Report, entitled *Danger at the Drug Store*, pharmacists are being blamed for drug-mix interactions that lead to injury or death. Although doctors prescribe these drugs, the report suggests that pharmacists are the last line of defense against risky drug interactions. In other words, after a person leaves the doctor's office with a handful of prescriptions, as most people usually do — if the doctor was not aware that two of the drugs that he prescribed produce harmful effects when taken together, the pharmacist must catch the error.

Additionally, if the physician forgets to warn the patients about the foods that must be avoided when taking the drug, then the pharmacist must catch that, too. Unfortunately, some pharmacists neglect to do this. They simply fill the prescriptions, and then send the person on his or her merry way. Several days later, they learn that the person was injured or resting in a morgue.

There are several reasons for this negligence. One is that the human factor is nearly absent in contemporary healthcare. The sadistic quest for profits in the healthcare industry has made it inhumane. As for doctors, many of them answer to HMO directors, whose only concern is the "bottom-line". The patient's needs are second-class.

This sentiment has spilled into the retail drug business. According to the report, the increasing financial turmoil in the retail drug business has many pharmacists working under greater stress. Mistakes are easily made when people are overworked and underpaid.

Food-to-drug interactions are also major concerns. When considering that certain foods can cause physical complications, it is reasonable that drugs mixed with foods can also cause harm. This subject was covered in an article entitled, *Some Food and Drugs Don't Mix*.[137] It is not surprising that some people are not aware of the foods that should be avoided when taking particular drugs. For that matter, drug makers and medical professionals are not aware, either. Again, it takes several hundred people to suffer or die before they become aware. Every drug coming from the pharmaceutical industry is experimental.

To date, many food-to-drug interactions have been identified. Many more have not. In one example, researchers learned that calcium channel blocking and anti-depressant drugs do not mix with grapefruit or grapefruit juice.[138] Grapefruit enhance the effects of these drugs, causing overdose.

Calcium channel blockers are used to treat high blood pressure by relaxing the blood vessels. This makes it easier for the heart to pump blood. When this effect is embellished two or three times over, life-threatening results occur. Likewise, overdosing on anti-depressant drugs can cause severe neuronal damage, leading to further mental conditions.

Another example is the adverse food-to-drug interaction of blood-thinning drugs, such as Coumadin. Persons taking this class of nostrums are warned to avoid natural blood-thinning elements, such as vitamin K. Vegetables such as broccoli, brussels sprouts, and cabbage contain vitamin K. These foods can block the effectiveness of this drug, bringing about life-threatening results, such as blood clots in the brain, lungs, and heart.

It appears that people using this drug are exempt from following the advice to eat more vegetables, specifically those vegetables rich in vitamin K. This presents another concern. People are required to exchange adequate nutrition for drug treatment. This does not make sense. The obvious result is poor health. This is partly the reason drugs are ineffective in solving chronic ailments.

Persons taking more than one medication, which happens to be many people nowadays, are at greater risk of drug-to-drug and drugs-to-foods adverse reactions. Some people have 4, 5, or 7 prescriptions. Their medical practitioners are having a field day.

Obesity Still Driving Drug Market

Despite the low efficacy of pharmaceuticals, and the dangers associated with using them, the demand for drugs is expected to grow. In the U.S., alone, pharmaceutical sales are expected to reach $330 billion by 2006.[139] To boot, the overweight and obese populations will continue to foot the larger load of these sales, as the use and cost of medications are markedly increased in obese populations.[140] Data shows that obese persons are greater consumers of medication for diabetes, cardiovascular disease, nonsteroidal anti-inflammatory and pain, and asthma. These drugs are sales leaders across the globe.

Surgical Procedures

From the outset, we must establish two logics or truths. First, whether we believe in Almighty God or not, we can all agree that none of us are the makers of our bodies. Our bodies come with the life force we have, neither of which we are consciously aware of until years after we are born.

Figure 9. Internal organs

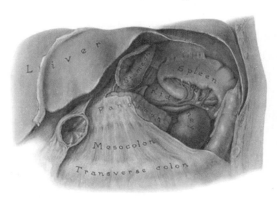

Therefore, not being the makers of our bodies, we must accept the fact that whoever made the human body had a purpose for every organ. Every organ has an important role. This leads to the second fact.

If the human body is disfigured in any way, such as through the removal or severing of an organ, then long-term consequences will definitely result. This is assured, and is a logical deduction. Therefore, we need not fool ourselves into thinking that there is no adverse health affect associated with the surgical manipulation of our bodies, particularly a bariatric surgical procedure — wherein organs to the life-sustaining digestive system are removed or severely altered.

Neither should we allow any medical practitioner to fool us into looking at the removal of any body organ in a light-hearted way. Once upon time, "bleeding" was viewed as an essential practice to curing diseases.[141] The thousands of people who suffered from this asinine and brutal treatment, many of which bled to death, confirmed the realization that blood was the fluid of life, and that losing too much of it spelled death. Today, blood banks are in need of blood to treat health ailments. No one is deliberately "bleeding" people to cure health problems.

In today's healthcare arena, people are not always fully informed about the long-term effects of surgical procedures. In other cases, medical practitioners are unaware of these, themselves, especially experimental procedures. Actually, the removal of any organ is an experimental procedure. It is through the results of medical experiments that health scientists are able to determine the efficacy of a treatment.

For example, early reports indicated that gastric procedures were free of long-term metabolic complications, but that has been retracted via post-surgery investigations. Neurological complications and micronutrient deficiencies are now associated with these operations. Scientists learned that there was a direct neurological line between the brain, stomach and intestines. Many patients suffered through this learning process. Consequently, some of the more invasive bariatric surgical procedures are no longer used.

The person undergoing the surgical procedure must be aware of the possible worst-case scenarios resulting from the surgery. They should also be aware that, although general side-effects are associated with surgeries, patients often have a specific cadre of these, as well as other side-effects, unique to them.

Rationale

Bariatric surgery proponents offer several rationales for this form of treatment. One is that this treatment is most effective for persons classified as morbidly obese. Morbid obesity correlates with a BMI of 40 kg/m², or with excessive weight of 100 or more pounds above the normal weight.

As previously discussed, being overweight is associated with increased morbidity and mortality from chronic diseases and other acute health ailments. For morbidly obese persons, the health risk is magnified. For example, the mortality rates for men 50% above average weight increases two-fold.[142] In this same weight group, the mortality increases five-fold for diabetics and four-fold for those with digestive tract disease.

In morbidly obese women, the mortality risk increases two-fold. And, in female diabetics, the risk increases eight-fold, and three-fold in those with digestive tract disease. Again, weight loss has been shown to decrease the overall health risks.

For the morbidly obese person, the issue regarding weight loss is whether dietary or behavioral modification treatments are feasible to reduce weight in time to stave off more severe health conditions, particularly death. With the person knocking at death's door, health officials have suggested surgical treatment is medically necessary because it is the only proven method of achieving long-term weight control for the morbidly obese.[143]

The overriding position is that bariatric surgery *"is a rationale supported by the time-honored principle that diseases which harm call for therapeutic intervention that, while vigorous, is less harmful than the disease being treated."*[144] This position, though reasonable, is highly debatable in the obesity context.

Bariatric surgery proponents have also spruced up the rationale for this procedure by contending that morbid obesity is a disease. Yet, they cite the same disturbances in appetite and hunger mechanisms that occur in the overweight or mildly obese person. Morbid obesity is overweight in its most serious and progressive state, but unless overweight can be called a disease, then morbid obesity cannot be classified as one.

Anatomical Consideration

Before reviewing the types of bariatric surgeries, their efficacy as an obesity treatment, and the adverse health consequences associated with them, let us review the workings of the stomach and intestine, two organs manipulated in bariatric surgeries.

The stomach is a temporary storage tank for food, where the initial chemical breakdown of food occurs. Therefore, when it comes to the manipulation of this organ, we must keep in mind that our stomachs are mathematically designed to serve its purpose, and that in this design, innate or intrinsic expectations are factored.

For example, the stomach's lining secretes a host of enzymes and hormones to aid digestion. Does the body know that this organ has been stapled or severed, and thereby, reduces the amount of digestive secretions? The complications associated with this particular aspect are detailed later in the next section.

Additionally, the stomach's gastric juices sanitize the food before it enters the small intestine. Immune cells are also located in the stomach and throughout the gastrointestinal tract.[145] Therefore, the cutting away of the stomach and small intestine impedes immunity, causing infections to easily occur.

Figure 10. Stomach [internal view]

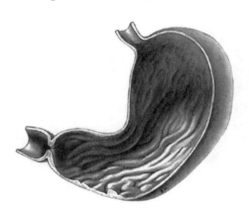

With respect to the small intestine, often called the bowel or gut, this organ is the major site of nutrient degradation and absorption. The intestinal lining releases many types of digestive enzymes and hormones to aid digestion. Other organs, such as the liver, releases substances into the gut. After the food is broken down in the intestine, it passes through into the bloodstream for use by the cells.

It should be obvious that when any part of the small intestine is severed, this entire process is significantly disturbed. A multitude of malabsorption and digestive problems ensue. Additionally, the body is not supplied the required nutrients. Other complications also develop.

Medical scientists have intensively studied the neuronal mechanisms of the gut. This study has yielded significant results. For one, scientists have learned that the intestine has its own nervous system — the *enteric* nervous system. It contains nerves connected to the central nervous system, as well as nerves independent of the central nervous system. The autonomic nervous system of the body is comprised of both central and enteric nervous systems.

Dr. Michael D. Gershon, in his book, *The Second Brain* states:[146]

> *We now know that there is a brain in the bowel, however inappropriate that concept might seem to be. The ugly gut is more intellectual than the heart and may have a greater capacity for "feeling". It is the only organ that contains an intrinsic nervous system that is able to mediate reflexes in the complete absence of input from the brain or spinal cord.*

Figure 11. Intestines

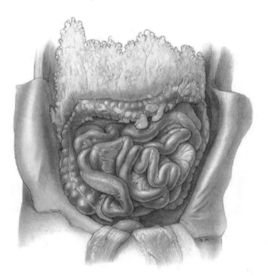

The intestine contains more than 100 million nerve cells, which is approximately equal to the number of nerve cells in the spinal cord. This system also contains scores of every class of neurotransmitters found in the brain — acetylcholine, noradrenaline, adrenaline, dopamine, glycine, y-aminobutyrate, glutamic acid, substance P, enkephalins, endorphins and serotonin.

In fact, 95% of the body's serotonin is made in the bowel. Knowing this, we can assume that any surgical manipulation to this organ cause adverse nervous conditions. This is precisely the case with bariatric surgery.

Common Surgical Procedures

Bariatric surgeries were common obesity treatments from the 1960's through the 1980's. Now, because of failed drug and dietary efforts, as well as the epidemic of "super obesity", these procedures are rapidly becoming popular. In the U.S., they have skyrocketed over the last decade, increasing 194% to 47,000 surgeries performed in 2001. This is up from 16,000 surgeries in 1992.[147]

Again, the rise in morbid obesity is partly responsible for this growth. Overweight persons are also opting for this surgery, although this treatment is not recommended for them.

Figure 12. Bariatric Surgery...Why?

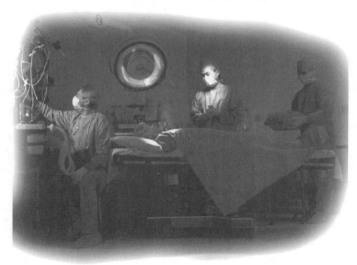

Bariatric surgeries are of several types, with the primary two being restrictive and gastric bypass. These procedures are less invasive than the outdated jejuno-ileal or intestinal bypass procedure, which caused severe nutrient deficiencies and liver disease.[116]

Gastric Restrictive

Gastric restrictive procedures include vertical banded gastroplasty (VBG), silastic ring gastroplasty (SRG) and adjustable silastic gastric banding (AGB). These procedures restrict the amount of food a person can eat at one setting by making the stomach smaller. In some cases, the size of the stomach is made small enough to only fit 0.5 to 1 cup of food before the person begins to feel uncomfortably full.

Figure 13. Stomach [abdomen view]

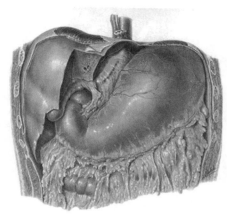

A scientific review of the success of restrictive procedures indicated that about 80% of patients lost some weight, and 30% reached their normal weight.[148] Three years after the operation, 50% of these people maintained the weight loss. After 10 years, this dropped to 26%.

The meager success of this procedure over the long-term is due to poor dietary practices. Discipline is still required to keep off the weight; otherwise, the constant eating will bring back the weight.

Hernia is the most common complication experienced by patients. Over one-third of patients develop gallstones. Between 10% and 20% of patients require subsequent surgeries to fix organ-related complications.

In addition, persistent vomiting may result, especially if the person keeps trying to eat more than the pouch can hold. This could also result in stretching the pouch, thereby, nullifying any benefit from the surgery.

It is also possible for the plastic band to wear through the stomach wall; thus causing the stomach to leak gastric juices into the abdominal cavity. This produces a serious infection called peritonitis.

Other complications of gastric restrictive procedures include abscess, fistulas, pulmonary embolism, low food intolerance, wound infections, band slippage, deep vein thrombosis, and pouch enlargement. Of course, there is always the risk of death.

Additionally, foods that contain little or no fiber, such as highly refined foods, move through the pouch more quickly than does wholesome foods, such as vegetables. This makes keeping a healthy diet challenging. This aspect, alone, is worth considering when deciding whether to have this surgery.

Gastric Bypass

In gastric bypass surgery, both the stomach and small intestine are altered. The small intestine is cut, and its lower part is connected to the small pouch, thereby, bypassing the lower stomach and the upper part of the small intestine.

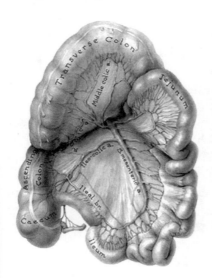

Figure 14. Superior Mesenteric

The objective of this surgical procedure is two-fold — reduce the stomach's storage capacity and reduce the absorption capacity of the small intestine. The most common gastric bypass surgery is called a *Roux-en-Y* gastric bypass.[149]

Health researchers have found greater weight loss in gastric bypass patients than with patients who underwent sole restrictive procedures.[150] Approximately two years after the surgery, patients have been shown to lose two-thirds of excess weight.[148] The success rate for weight loss is 68% to 72% of excess over a three year period.[151] After five years, the average weight loss ranges from 48% to 74%.[144]

In a gastric bypass, the part of the intestine where many minerals and vitamins are most easily absorbed is bypassed. Because of this, patients become deficient in iron, calcium, magnesium, and other vitamins. This can lead to long-term problems, such as osteoporosis. To prevent vitamin and mineral deficiencies, patients must take nutrient supplements or injections of vitamins.

As with restrictive procedures, hernia is the most common complication; approximately one-third of patients develop gallstones; and about 20% also require subsequent surgeries to repair complications. Peritonitis may also develop. In addition, many patients develop liver problems.

Other risks associated with major surgery include infection in the incision, an abscess inside the abdomen, deep vein thrombosis, and pulmonary embolism. There is a greater risk of death associated with this procedure, as about 1 in 2,000 (0.5%) persons die. Table 5 lists the type of complications associated with bariatric surgeries.

Table 5: Complications Associated with Bariatric Surgery

So-called Minor	So-called Major
• Atelectasis, hyperventilation, other respiratory conditions	• GI Leak
• wound site seroma, wound infection	• stoma obstruction (lumenal); stoma stenosis
• splenic injury	• GI hemorrhage or GI bleeding
• pleural effusion, pleuritis, and pneumonitis	• cardiac
• dehydration	• pulmonary embolism
• renal, urinary tract infection	• respiratory arrest or failure
• stoma too large, stoma too small	• wound dehiscence
• ulcers (duodenal, gastric, stomal)	• small bowel obstruction
• hepatic, liver hematoma	• subphrenic, subhepatic, abdominal abscess
• esophageal reflux, esophagitis	• gastric dilatation
• hernia	• deep venous thrombosis, thrombophlebitis
• dumping syndrome, vitamin insufficiency	• stapleline breakdown
	• pancreatitis, acute cholecystitis
	• gastric fistula
	• peritonitis

In one of the most comprehensive reports about the complications of bariatric surgeries, approximately 11,000 bariatric patients were assessed.[152] Females comprised 84.3% of patients, and 15.7% were male. The patient's body mass index at operation was 49.1 kg/m2. The mean-age of the patients was 39.8 years.

The report evaluated complications that occurred within 30 days following surgical treatment. The types of operations varied according to surgeon recommendation, procedure availability, and patient choice. The operations, however, were divided according to complexity and not according to the type of surgery performed. Complex operations included combination gastric restriction and gastric bypass procedures. Simple procedures included gastric restriction only. Overall, 79% of the operations were complex.

Here, we must note that 97% of the procedures performed in 2000 were complex, compared to 11.5% in 1986. This means the persons undergoing bariatric procedures can expect to deal with both short-term and long-term complications.

One exploratory study examined the occurrence of duodenogastric bile reflux to the excluded stomach after Roux-en-Y gastric bypass. This study showed that in more than one third of the gastric bypass patients, the gastric mucosa in the excluded stomach is exposed to the potential deleterious effects of bile.[148] Again, how do the organs that release digestive substances into the stomach and intestine know that these organs have been severed or altered? They do not, so the continue to do their job in *business as usual* fashion.

Surgical obesity treatment, although claiming to lower obesity-related medication costs, increases other medication costs.[135] The person experiences no cost savings. As noted, complications of the surgery are life-long, requiring life-long treatment. This means life-long expenditures.

Consider This

Perhaps the principle consideration with respect to the need for bariatric surgery is whether the correct diet for human adults have been tried. For many, it has not been tried. Very few know about it. The evil forces that desire profits have effectively covered this dietary guidance by misrepresenting to the people those who represent this divine dietary guidance. This guidance, however, is addressed in Chapter 6.

People must resolve the core issues about diet — the proper foods humans should eat and how often these foods should be eaten to achieve excellent health and longevity. We also address this in the forthcoming chapters.

Holistic Remedies

Holistic remedies, particularly herbal products and supplements, have been used to treat obesity.[154] These products are part of the nutraceutical market, which is not regulated by the FDA.

Being unregulated, the vast majority of herbal products are deficient in appropriate human toxicological analysis. And, because they are considered all natural, and therefore safe, these concoctions are abused and overused. Quackery is at its best in this unregulated industry.

Like their counterparts, so-called holistic remedies have rang up a toll of suffering and death. For example, in 1994, Jin Bu Huan herbal tablets, sold as sedatives, were directly linked to cases of severe liver toxicity in both adults and children. In 1992, the FDA warned several health food store chains to stop distributing dietary supplements containing gum guar after numerous cases of esophageal obstruction were linked to the use of these products. Recently, deaths resulting from *ma-huang* or *ephedra* in adolescents and young adults forced the FDA to render restraints on the unethical advertising practices used by manufacturers of these products.

In addition to injury, people are ripped off when purchasing many of these products. In one study, the 10 most commonly purchased herbs were tested to see if what was written on the label was, in fact, contained in the pills.[155] Products for each of 10 herbs were surveyed in a convenience sample of 20 retail stores in a large metropolitan area. The products selected were those that had the greatest sales dollars in 1998. These were echinacea, St. John's wort, Ginkgo biloba, garlic, saw palmetto, ginseng, goldenseal, aloe, Siberian ginseng, and valerian.

Each herb had a large range in label ingredients and recommended daily dose (RDD). Among 880 products, 43% were consistent with a benchmark in ingredients and RDD. Approximately, 20% were consistent in ingredients only.

In another study, the famous herb, St. John's Wort, was on the witness stand.[156] This herb is primarily used to treat mild depression. Concern about the purity and content of commercial preparations was an impetus for this study.

Fifty-four St. John's wort products were purchased in Canada and in the U.S. They were analyzed for the two active ingredients that make the product effective. Only two products had concentrations of ingredients within 10% of the label claim. Some contained none of the active ingredients. On average, there was half the amount of claimed ingredients.

We reiterate the fact that ingesting many various chemicals and foods puts us in harm's way. People, generally, place too much crap into their bodies, believing that good health will be the outcome. To expect an herbal remedy to overcome the toxins caused by eating bad foods and by eating food too often is an irrational expectation. This will not happen.

Consider This

The objective of this world's treatments for obesity is clear — to make profit. And, if perchance, there are sincere medical practitioners who offer these bogus treatments, the essential questions surrounding diet, nutrition and health must still be answered. These questions are:

1. *What foods are fit for humans to eat?*

2. *How often should humans eat these foods?*

The answers to these questions serve as the foundation for diet and nutrition education. They also represent two pillars of longevity. In the next chapter, this vital information is addressed.

CHAPTER 6

Divine Guidance

Throughout the books, *How To Eat To Live*, the cause of illness and disease is made very plain. Our mismanagement of food brings about disease. This includes the types of foods eaten, how they are prepared, and how often we eat them. The cause of diseases is far less complicated than the solutions promoted by industries whose aim is to make profit.

The U.S. Department of Health and Human Services also points to improper diet as the cause of disease. In the document, *Healthy People 2000 Review 1995-96*, it states:

> *Dietary factors contribute substantially to preventable illness and premature death in the United States. For the majority of Americans who do not smoke and do not drink excessively, what they eat is the most significant controllable risk factor affecting their long-term health. Five major causes of death are associated with dietary factors: coronary heart disease, some types of cancer, stroke, noninsulin-dependent diabetes mellitus, and coronary artery disease.*

Additionally, the efforts of this world's heath scientists and practitioners are to treat obesity, and not prevent it. No prevention strategy exists. The following is from an article entitled, *Prevention of obesity - is it possible?*[157]

> *Obesity prevention is necessary to address the steady rise in the prevalence of obesity. Although all experts agree that obesity prevention has high priority, there is almost no research in this area. There is also no structured framework for obesity prevention. The effectiveness of different intervention strategies is not well documented.*

The reasons for this lack of prevention efforts have been delineated. In Chapter 1, we established the deceptive ploy of the problem/failed-solution recycling process, particularly the continuous recycling of obesity-related dietary advice, articles, reports, epidemiological studies, medicines, nostrums and fact-finding commissions.

The framework of this recycling process is a system of deception, which is supported by the ever-degenerating state of fallen-man. This state is widespread evil permeating from a mindset that has the goal of fulfilling every vain and low desire. The only variables are the severity of the problems, and the players (victims and culprits). The conditions worsen because the degenerative state of the human mind worsens, morally deteriorating day-by-day.

There are several dynamics that drive this recycling process; however, the root factor is the absence of or disobedience to divine guidance. One might ask, *what does the obesity epidemic have to do with Almighty God, the Scriptures and religion?* It has everything to do with them. The same goes for the multitude of other epidemics that have gripped the human family.

In this world, where make-believe, fantasies, and fairytales reign supreme, the things of God are relegated to ignorant and empty religious rituals and practice that most people find unsuitable and impossible to apply in their daily living. This is because they are precisely that — unsuitable and impossible, plus impertinent, baseless, and ridiculous, to boot.

The fairytales we learn as children, such as the "cow jumping over the moon", extend through adulthood in religious thought and practice. The way we are taught to view the things of God cannot serve our needs, any more than the concept of the "cow jumping over the moon" can help us obtain food, clothing and shelter.

Guidance is direction or advice as to a decision or course. As humans, each of us is on the journey to achieve that which we are born to do. Divine guidance, therefore, is the direction from Almighty God that leads us to the fulfillment of our purpose for existing. Such guidance is not relegated to song-n-dance, choirs, musical instruments, and other elements of showmanship that comprise traditional religious expression. Unfortunately, these things are the hallmark of today's religious practice. Little to no guidance of divine living is offered. Most people stagger through life, while claiming to be saved. Yet, they ultimately are not *saved* from the evil ploys that robbed them of money and life.

As with any journey, decisions must be made along the way. Mandates, recommendations, and advice are offered to aid the journey. All of this affects and involves every aspect of human life and living. In fulfilling our purpose for living, a true relationship with Almighty God, as well as essential interpersonal relationships must be established and upheld through appropriate responsibility and accountability.

Additionally, good health must be maintained, because sickness and disease threatens life, thus threatening the journey. It is our responsibility to not become "willing" burdens to our loved ones by acting negligent toward our health.

Therefore, divine guidance does not leave any stone unturned in instructing humans about the best way to live. These stones include diet, domestic living, business matters, government systems, and every conceivable relationship that one has with other people and with the environment. Divine guidance, when accepted, produces civilization.

Evidence that divine guidance is being followed is the pervasiveness of righteousness, loving families, peace, happiness, contentment, and long, healthy life spans. Where on this earth are such conditions found? Almost not anywhere! And, although people might call these heavenly conditions fantasy, they represent the environment that Almighty God intends for human life. Therefore, not living this grand life is an indictment against the present world, rather than a figment of a righteous person's imagination.

Yet, some people will mock a person for believing that such a blissful society or world is achievable. This demonstrates the fallen state of the human psyche. That great, good, and pure things can happen in today's society is becoming the remotest of all thoughts.

Divine guidance also evolves, because it comprises those instructions that enable humans to transcend the contemporary plagues of evil and ignorance that produces the destructive conditions under which they live. Yesterday's divine revelation is not sufficient to solve today's disastrous human plight, of which the obesity pandemic is a part.

This fact is demonstrated in the obesity epidemic, itself, as Christians, Jews and Muslims are under this burden, in spite of the divine dietary laws they have through the Gospel, Torah, and Holy

Quran, respectively. Obesity has spread to all corners of the globe, afflicting humans regardless of race, creed, or color.[14] According to the World Health Organization, obesity rates have risen three-fold or more since 1980 in North America, the United Kingdom, Eastern Europe, the Middle East, the Pacific Islands, Australia and China.[15] Every creed is practiced in these lands.

For example, one epidemiological study confirmed obesity as a greater health risk in the Middle East than in other parts of the world.[158] In 2001, researchers estimated that 23% of the United Arab Emirates population were obese. The estimate of obesity in Kuwait was a staggering 49%. In addition, the greatest concern was not the obesity prevalence, but the poor awareness of the obesity crisis in the Middle East. Researchers claimed that these populations were ignorant about obesity prevention and intervention methods. So, it appears that other guidance is necessary over-and-above simply abstaining from swine flesh, as God commands Believers to do.

Health researchers admit to a lack of effective treatment options for reducing the obesity pandemic. They implore that fighting obesity requires an effective population-based strategy that includes conceptual shifts and the participation of key systemic institutions — education, politics, health, business, and all other institutions that affect and determine one's quality of life.[120] Bringing these institutions into a cohesive strategy under this type of governing system, where greed is the overriding aim, is fantasy.

Revisiting the dark-age context, we reexamine this quote by Marc Widdowson:

> *The dark age is a melting pot when the old, corrupt and exhausted institutions that we have long outgrown are finally broken down and destroyed. Then something new and better suited to human needs can gradually be built up in their place.*

There is much in this. Today, most of us know that nearly every system associated with the so-called contemporary way of life is failing. Many of these systems have already completely failed. The magnificent buildings, landscapes, and technologies out of which these institutions and systems operate fool many people into believing that these systems are serving our needs.

However, that which is produced from these institutions shows that they have long failed. The products of these institutions, including human beings via the educational and religious systems; policies and laws via the political system; and medical care via the healthcare system, continuously add fuel to a fire that has long been out of control. These institutions have died a certain death because they are, in fact, *old, corrupt,* and *exhausted* — unable to provide the citizenry with the quality of life Almighty God wants for His creation.

Be it unknown to many, something new is gradually supplanting the systems that support the bogus way of living manufactured for us by the *comfortable beneficiaries.* That something is the "life" that Almighty God ordained for humans to live. There are very identifiable proofs that reveal how such a life is gradually being given to humanity. Among these identifiable proofs is the extraordinary pain that nearly everyone is now experiencing.

Mr. Widdowson continues:

> *For the comfortable beneficiaries of the old institutions, this is exclusively a painful process. For all the rest, who are far more numerous, it is painful but also hopeful.*

This pain is extraordinary because it is not only caused by adherence to the death-dealing, criminal machinations of the evildoers that take our money and lives away. This pain is unbearably intensified through the spread of truth and the rise of the truth givers.

This truth expels falsehood in the minds of the people, while dismantling a world system that totally relies on falsehood in order to flourish. Because falsehood is not reality, anything built on it is only an illusion, and vanishes in the light of truth. If this falsehood happens to be an educational system, then when truth comes, the inept and savage behaviors of past and present students are exposed, as an indictment against this world's educational system.

It is this expelling or vanquishing of falsehood that brings on this intense pain. Because the truth represents the arrival of another world — a world based on divine living — the *comfortable beneficiaries* of the old and corrupt institutions experience a painful demise. Yet, they do not give in without a fight. Moreover, they use everything at their disposal to challenge the New Thought and those who carry it. Their ultimate aim is to destroy the truth givers. Slander is among the many tactics used by the *comfortable beneficiaries* to wage war against the New Order.

In spite of their efforts to slander and destroy the truth givers, they fail. They also are disgraced in the process, before the deathblow is dealt to their world. They end up ruined and ostracized.

They fail because the hurling of the truth into the minds of the people is not overcome. Again, because this truth is Almighty God's divine guidance, in action, people are attracted to it, in varying levels. This Guidance contains the magnetic force that, initially, causes a mental imbalance, as the people are forced to compare it against everything they have been taught by the *comfortable beneficiaries*. This mental imbalance gradually levels out as we begin to order our lives according to the truth.

The truth forces a decision — do we continue in error or clean up? Either we make a decision or go further into insanity. In this context, insanity becomes a price of indecision. No doubt, the wrong decision exacerbates the insanity.

We can only wonder what kind of person would opt out of a plan that insures longevity and true prosperity in exchange for a painful and premature demise at the hands of the *comfortable beneficiaries*. Unfortunately, too many people are in this group. They have grown in love with self-destruction.

Let us briefly examine the methodologies employed by the *comfortable beneficiaries* to maintain the *old*, *corrupt* and *exhausted* institutions that have long failed. To preface this, let us consider the following.

To date, much ado is made about healthcare. Is acquiring good health supposed to be evasive? Did the Creator intend humans to have to dole out trillions of dollars for healthcare services? Most of us can agree that God's intent was not for us to spend these inordinate efforts and resources to maintain good health.

The first man and woman, called Adam, had no healthcare facility to cater to their needs. They had a divine way of living, complete with a garden and a dietary law. These were suitable to enable the Old Biblical patriarchs, Noah and Methuselah, to have life spans of hundreds of years. How is it now that most people can hardly live 100 years, and to live this meager span, much money is spent for medicines, surgeries and other health services? We are deceived.

So now, what are the *comfortable beneficiaries* methodologies of deception? On the surface, it is a three-fold scheme. First, they must dumb-down the population through the promotion of lies, fantasies and fairytales. The peoples' minds must become lands of "make-believe". Commonsense must become a casualty. This makes the people amenable to falling for anything, no matter how silly, ridiculous, and farfetched. Worst, this extraordinary dumbing-down makes people treat truth as falsehood and falsehood as truth.

Secondly, the *comfortable beneficiaries* must confuse issues of importance because this affords them the greatest opportunity to extract wealth from the population. What is more important to each of us than our health? Therefore, if the quest to obtain and maintain good health is made obscure and confusing, various schemes can be launched to snatch money away from us. The obesity issue is a prime example. As we have learned, gross confusion surrounds this problem, in every respect.

Finally, the *comfortable beneficiaries* must make the truth and the truth-givers — those who represent that "*something new and better suited to human needs*" — appear to the people other than what they really are. They must make the good the truth-givers do appear evil. They must also detract the peoples' attention from the truth by slandering the truth-givers.

In doing this, the *comfortable beneficiaries* of these worthless institutions believe that the truth will become a casualty. They are wrong. They are also hypocritical, which seals their doom even more. This hypocrisy is shown in their use of the truth, and this New Knowledge, to elevate themselves in their faltering society. So, while they attempt to eliminate the truth-givers, as well as certain aspects of the truth, they take bits and pieces of this truth to advance themselves. They never admit to nor reveal the whole truth.

One example of this is demonstrated in how the *comfortable beneficiaries* portray the Teaching of the Honorable Elijah Muhammad. In general, the population's knowledge of the Teachings is, primarily, relegated to the knowledge given about the origin of the Caucasian race. Even this portrait is tainted by the evildoers. Because of their mischief-making through the media, most people erroneously and ignorantly call this knowledge "hate" teachings.

Nevertheless, too few people are aware of the great body of scientific, mathematical and societal knowledge the Honorable Elijah Muhammad taught; and that Minister Louis Farrakhan and those who follow him continue to teach. This is the reason both men are greatly misunderstood by the public, yet this knowledge absolutely represents a new paradigm for every area of human life.

It is only when people are given the opportunity to hear these men for themselves that they understand them better and appreciate the body of knowledge these two men and those who follow them possess. Unfortunately, these opportunities are frustrated, curtailed, or misrepresented by the *comfortable beneficiaries*, who control the mass media. They continue to sell the people on old, outdated and slanderous fallacies.

Careful examination of this world's scientific explosion reveals that it was and is rooted in the Teachings of the Honorable Elijah Muhammad. This is also illustrated in the dietary arena. For example, let us examine the back cover of the books, *How To Eat To Live*. Figure 15 shows this cover.

Everything written on this cover is verifiable, with little effort. As for the next to the last statement, there are several reasons why the *comfortable beneficiaries* have taken the Honorable Elijah Muhammad's teachings about diet, and convoluted it by mixing in falsehoods. Again, the foremost reason is that the food and medical industries are commercial industries, and therefore, are profit-driven.

How much money would a dietary law that curtails food expenditures, lessens doctor visitations, abolishes the need for prescription drugs, and halts the consumption of divinely-prohibited foods that currently generate billions of dollars, cost these industries? What impact would a revolutionary change to the populations' dietary practices have on this nation's pocketbook? The impact would be tremendous. It would nearly collapse the economy.

Even with this borrowing of divine guidance, the *comfortable beneficiaries* leave much out. Yes, because of the Honorable Elijah Muhammad's teachings, wheat bread has become the most popular bread to eat. Yes, fruits and vegetables also are preferred over processed foods. Yes, people are encouraged to reduce their intake of meat. Nonetheless, the merchants of death continue to keep divinely-prohibited foods and drinks, swine flesh and alcohol, in the marketplace. They also continue to promote gluttony of both good and bad foods.

Figure 16. Back cover of How To Eat To Live

The Teachings of Muhammad

For more than 30 years, Messenger Elijah Muhammad has been teaching the so-called Negroes of America on the proper foods to eat to improve their mental power, physical appearance, for prevention of illness, curing of ailments and prolonging life.

Before it became a fad, Messenger Muhammad advocated eating whole wheat and staying away from bleached, white enriched flour. He has taught and maintained fats should be reduced and eliminated from the diet. He has warned about the dangers of eating from cans and wax cartons. He has cautioned the so-called Negroes to take better care in selecting food to eat.

Mr. Muhammad has stated the so-called Negro should eat the young, fresh green vegetables. He has stated the lima bean, black-eyed peas and other field beans do not have food values good for the body and that they are very hard and damaging to the digestive tract.

For more than 30 years, the Muslim home has stressed the baking of foods and not frying. He has cautioned his followers to be conscious of weight. Penalties are exacted from Muslims found overweight.

All of Messenger Muhammad's teaching on foods and weight have been studied by white scientists, doctors and dieticians. Finally, 1959, actuaries released new average weight charts for men and women. It was no mere coincidence that their findings coincide with what Messenger Muhammad had been teaching. It was practically a verbatim transcript of the papers they confiscated when the federal government arrested him in 1942.

This was followed up with a featured story on weight in the "U.S. News & Word Report," Nov. 2, 1959, which was condensed in "Reader's Digest," Feb, 1960. Their story, too, followed what Messenger Muhammad has been teaching for 30 years, that is, except the portions which advise eating pork, "Coronet" magazine, also in Feb., 1960, published an article on weight and new weight charts, according to the plan of Mr. Muhammad. And, in the April 11, 1960 edition, the "U.S. News & World Report" again reported a detailed account on the foods to eat. As one Muslim said, "They really listened to Mr. Muhammad, but they mixed it up and added to it." Everyone would do well to read this book by Mr. Muhammad on the proper foods to eat. His advice adds to your life.

****

As Truth cannot be purchased, this book is a gift to you in exchange for your contribution which will be used to build a much needed educational center for Black men in Chicago.

May God bless every purchaser of this book.

(Reprinted from original cover, 1972)

This re-print is under the auspices of Minister Louis Farrakhan and the Nation of Islam, National Center, 7531 So. Stony Island Ave., Chicago, IL 60620 1-773-602-1230

Disease/Solution

Generally, through the Honorable Elijah Muhammad, humanity has been given the knowledge of Almighty God's value of life — the life He has created. In the Scriptures, Almighty God clearly demonstrates His interest in the affairs of humans. In doing so, we learn that He brings from the earth that which man needs to properly nourish his body. He also tells man the precise foods to eat, and those to avoid.

How To Eat To Live is Almighty God's up-to-date dietary guidance for the human family. This guidance not only reminds us of the divine dietary mandates given in the Holy Quran and Bible, but also we are given the best teaching and instruction to protect our lives from the wiles of the *merchants of death, comfortable beneficiaries, evildoers, or Satan.*

In this Teaching, we have been given more information about food, food preparation, and diet than at anytime before - at least, the span of time covered in the Scriptures. No one should doubt that we need detailed guidance, today. The human family is clearly confused about diet. We have taken more despicable things as food than at anytime in the history of man.

Humans now eat nearly every creature on the earth, such as bugs, cats, dogs, eels, reptiles, monkey brains, feces and wild plants and bushes, to name a few. We also fed these things through the foods we eat, as the *merchants of death* place the body parts and scraps of animals into the foods many people eat.

In addition, mainstream or this world's dietary guidance has its base in gluttony. This point cannot be emphasized enough. Nutritionists advise the eating of fruits and vegetables three to five times a day, or they state very little about meal-time frequency, altogether. The consensus among them, however, is that adults should eat more than once a day. Again, where is the medical research that substantiates the eating of three or more meals a day as the means of achieving good health? There is none.

Cause of Sickness

The Honorable Elijah Muhammad, through his books *How To Eat To Live*, set our expectations for health and life by stating that there was no set time for us to die. Of course, no one lives forever, but the context of this statement is with respect to the short lives and short life expectancy people currently have. Scientists agree that the life's cell is made to continuously reproduce and regenerate, and that our false way of living prematurely ends these life-sustaining processes.[159]

We die when we fail to properly maintain the life force within our bodies. This position is supported by science. We wear our organs out through poor diets and reckless living, and the body cannot take that type of abuse and hold the life force.

Consequently, as our organs wear, they begin to fail. This failure is called by many names (for example, heart, kidney, liver, blood, and brain diseases). Many authors of health books spend thousands of pages describing these diseases and how to treat them. Although many of these books are sold, good health still evades the readers of these books, because the root cause is never addressed.

In *How To Eat To Live*, the Honorable Elijah Muhammad does not waste time naming diseases. He does not waste time describing *this* or *that* disease apart from its root. If the root is in diet, then that is the place to start. He does this in a simplistic, yet revolutionary way by pointing out the wrong foods we eat, and by showing us how eating food too often causes disease.

Logically, eating wrong foods and eating any food too often destroys health. His solution is also simple: eat one meal every 24 hours, of the right foods. This is the minimal dietary prescription for adults. For better health, we can eat our meals every 48 or 72 hours, if our livelihood allows us to do so. Please read the details of foods to eat and foods to avoid in the books, *How To Eat To Live*. And, for scientific support for this guidance, please read *FAQs About How To Eat To Live (Vol. 1 & 2)*, and *Nuts Are Not Good for Humans*, by this author.

The Honorable Elijah Muhammad states that 95% of our sickness comes from eating before we are hungry. We put the stomach to work before it calls for food. This statement indicates that there is a higher order in effect that makes the stomach or digestive system ready to receive food. Receiving something before we are ready for it can cause problems. Preparation is an intrinsic part of every human endeavor.

Eating before we are hungry causes a shock to the digestive system and entire body. This shock can be viewed as an extra and unnecessary blow to an already overtaxed body. The body is forced to handle a burden that it is not prepared to deal with — the awesome task of digesting more food. In most cases, the digestive system is already dealing with the meal or meals currently in its system, and to have more stuff thrown in it is overwhelming. To make this point clearer, let us briefly examine the digestive process.

Natural Operation of the Human Digestive System

We have learned that self-preservation is a law of nature. Some have said it is the first law of nature. It holds true that after life is granted, the ultimate responsibility is to maintain it as long as one can because death is the irrevocable will of the Creator. The chronic disease pandemic reveals that we know very little about preserving the only life each of us definitely know we will have.

Of course, merely knowing that *self-preservation is the law of nature* means little. The "how" to preserve it is the most important challenge.

One definition of preservation is:

The act or process of preserving, or keeping safe; the state of being preserved, or kept from injury, destruction, or decay; security; safety; as, preservation of life, fruit, game, etc.

Now, if self-preservation is a law of nature, it means that in the nature of the human being is the law or process of self-preservation. The body is, therefore, made to function in a way that preserves it. This means the body is self-governed in its biological operation. The workings of the autonomic nervous system and the many biological feedback systems that support the body prove that self-preservation is innate. We do not have to think about these processes. They just continue to function.

In fact, the scientific studies of weight gain demonstrate that the body is self-governed. However, this automation does not include the type of food we eat. The human being, using his or her God-given *free will* and intelligence, has the responsibility of putting the right foods into the body, in accordance with the way the body is created to operate. The quality of the food we eat and how often we eat it are among the few core variables that can disturb the innate biological processes.

Again, the chronic disease and early mortality pandemics show that our decisions have not been in accordance with the law of self-preservation. At the root of our wrong decisions is the lack of true knowledge about diet or rebellion against that truth. Because the *comfortable beneficiaries* of the *old, corrupted* and *exhausted* institutions of this world have deceived us for profit's sake, we can claim ignorance. In the onward march to protect our lives, we now must learn divine guidance.

As with anything made or created, the first place to go to learn how to maintain it is to the source — the person or thing that made or created it. Fortunately, for humans, only one source is responsible for our creation. And, although this subject opens up fierce debate and controversy, a scientific investigation of the biological workings of the human body is sufficient to support divine guidance and substantiate the best diet for humans.

Digestive Process

The digestive process is the means by which the nutrients required for the maintenance of the body, particularly the cell, are made available through the food we eat. To achieve this task, there are specific organs responsible for facilitating the digestive process. They make up the digestive system.

Basically, the digestive system is a hollow tube or tract that begins at the mouth and extends to the anus. Organs of the digestive tract or alimentary canal consist of the mouth, pharynx, esophagus, stomach, small intestine, and large intestines.

The accessory digestive organs that aid in this process include the salivary glands, gall bladder, liver, and pancreas. These organs assist in the digestive process by secreting substances that breakdown or emulsify food components. Working on concert with each other, these organs are responsible for food ingestion, digestion, absorption, and the elimination of the indigestible remains, called feces.

The main purpose of the digestion is to degrade food into its necessary components so that the biological cells can utilize them. The cell is considered the basic unit of life. Cells reproduce to make up tissues; and tissues make up organs; and organs give us the human body. Through it all, it is the biological cell that needs the material and energy to handle its vital processes.

Food is degraded by both mechanical means, such as chewing and churning; and by chemical means — through digestive enzymes that break the bonds of the molecules that compose the food. The digestive tract can be viewed as a "disassembly line".

The major nutrients of food that require digestion are proteins, starches, and fats. These large molecules are degraded into smaller units or their basic building blocks. Proteins are degraded to amino acids; starch, a polysaccharide is broken down into monosaccharides or simple sugars; and fats are degraded into smaller units, as well. These degraded nutrients are absorbed into the body system and used by the cells.

Figure 17. Digestive System

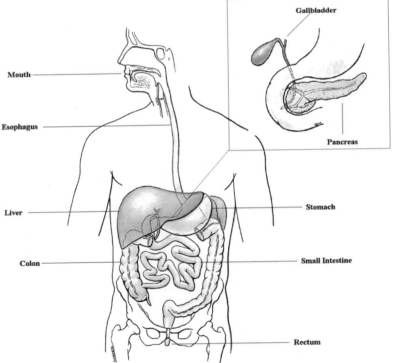

We must note that not all of these nutrients are degradable by the human digestive system, although they may be carbohydrates, proteins, and lipids (fats). It depends on food. Certain foods are composed of complex types of these substances, which our digestive organs and enzymes cannot process. The way these nutrients are bound determines their digestibility — whether our digestive enzymes can break them down.

We simply may not possess the organs and enzymes required to degrade this vegetation. This is the case with protease inhibitors and goitrogens, as previously discussed. In the end, we must reconcile that although certain indigestible foods taste good, they are fit for other creatures and not us.

These complex molecules can only be digested by animals that have the appropriate enzymes or gut microbial. This is why such terms — proteins, lipids, and carbohydrates — should never be used in a general sense when assessing the nutritional benefits of a particular food. The quality of these nutrients should be taken into account. This may require a new nomenclature for food science and labeling. Now back to the digestive process.

Our tongues and teeth, as well as specific digestive enzymes, begin the digestive process. For example, salivary amylase is an enzyme that starts the chemical digestion of starch, which, among other purposes, permits us to enjoy the taste of the food on our palates.

After the food is thoroughly chewed and mixed with saliva, it is pushed into the pharynx, and passes through the esophagus — the act of swallowing. At this point, the food is termed, *food bolus*. This is a clog of chewed food mixed with saliva. It no longer resembles the food that entered the mouth a short time, ago. To others, who may be at the dinner table, that food was more appealing before entering the mouth, so talking with food in your mouth can be offensive.

Peristaltic contractions move the food through the esophagus until it enters the stomach. While in the stomach, the food bolus is in the most hostile environment of the entire trip. It under goes a great deal of churning and mixing movements, while being acted upon by an array of chemicals that turns the bolus into a substance called, *chyme*.

Once chyme is produced, peristalsis begins in the lower half of the stomach and forces the chyme through an opening (pyloric sphincter) that leads to the duodenum. The duodenum is the first subdivision of the small intestines.

The passage of chyme into the small intestines is regulated to avoid an overflow of the duodenum; thus, only small amounts can enter at a time. It takes approximately 4 hours for the stomach to completely empty chyme into the small intestines. Of course, the actual time depends upon several factors. These factors include the digestibility of the food, the appropriate mastication of it, and the overall condition of the digestive tract.

The Honorable Elijah Muhammad emphasizes the point about properly masticating our food. Some people can finish off a huge plate of food in less than ten minutes, because they practically gulp down the food, hardly using their teeth. They throw the food down into their stomachs, and let the delicate digestive system do the heavy labor. They have no patience when eating. An array of health ailments is associated with this savage way of eating.

It is in the small intestines where food digestion is accelerated. The pancreas, liver, and gall bladder simultaneously release their digestive juices into the small intestines. The pancreatic juice contains enzymes that digest proteins, carbohydrates, fats, (and nucleic acids). The small intestine also releases its own digestive juices.

Figure 18. Liver [inferior/posterior view]

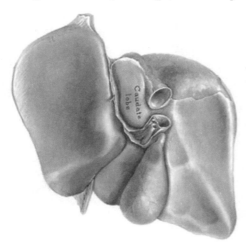

The liver and gall bladder releases bile into the small intestines. Bile is not an enzyme. It emulsifies or mechanically breaks down large fat molecules, which produces the appropriate surface for the fat-digesting enzyme, lipase, to work. Bile also has other important functions, such as assisting with the absorption of fat-soluble vitamins (K, A, and D).

If either bile or the pancreatic juices are absent, then essentially no fat digestion or absorption takes place. Among the many troubles that result is blood clotting. This is because the liver needs vitamin K to make a substance called *prothrombin*, which is a clotting factor.

The end-products of digestion — amino acids, monosaccharides, and fats — are absorbed throughout the small intestines into the blood stream. After passing through the filtering system or kidneys, these nutrients are available for use by the cells.

The small intestines are approximately ten feet in length. The chyme undergoes a 4 to 8 hour journey through this organ, and by the time the food finishes this course, the digestive process is nearly complete.

Finally, undigested material enters the large intestines. Although this material consists of residue, with few nutrients, it remains in the large intestines for approximately 12 hours. Essentially, no digestion takes place in the large intestines, except for digestive activity by bacteria that live there.

This bacterium also produces several vitamins (K and B). These vitamins, along with most of the remaining water, and some ions are absorbed through the large intestinal lining. After this, the waste materials or feces are delivered to the rectum for elimination.

If we add up the hours involved in the digestive process — 4 hours for stomach activity; up to 8 hours in the small intestines; and 12 hours in the large intestines — we see that food digestion is an important and time-consuming process. We also see that a total of 24 hours is required to completely digest a meal. Some reference materials, such as the *Encyclopedia of Human Biology*, state that it takes 40 to 60 hours for a meal to digest. Likewise, the Honorable Elijah Muhammad stated that it takes 36 hours to digest some foods.

Dietary Restriction

We can safely agree that it takes approximately 24 hours for a meal to be properly digested. Therefore, eating one meal a day is scientifically justified. Of course, following this restricts us against eating all day and all night. For the common person, such a revolutionary concept is new, and perhaps unbelievable. For some health scientists, this concept is not new. In fact, it is older than many people living today are.

Scientific investigations have long supported that eating less food produces healthier and longer life.[160] They call this eating process *dietary restriction*. Such a characterization implies that a person must have limits to his or her dietary habits. This is true. After all, if there are things that humans should not eat for health's sake, then these things should be restricted from our diets. Additionally, there must be some restriction to how often we eat and for the amount of food we eat.

Studies on dietary restriction date back more than 70 years. Several study models have been employed. For example, in some studies animals were allowed to eat ad libitum for a restricted amount of time, such as 12 hours every other day. In other studies, the animals were fed a certain amount of food that represented between 40% to 70% reduction of what they normally ate.

In one study concerning the effects of dietary restriction on diabetes, *Psammomys Obesus* (sand rats) were fed high-energy dense diets until they developed type II diabetes.[161] This particular animal was used because it was able to develop the disease in the same way humans develop it — through diet. Additionally, a high-energy dense diet was used because this diet causes obesity and diabetes.

There were many positive points in this study, but we will only note several. First, the animals were subjected to a two-week dietary program that not only included a reduction in food intake, but also featured a regulated daily feeding. They received a ration of food at 5 p.m. each day.

Although tests were not administered to the animals until after they ate ad libitum for two weeks following the restricted diet, the results were still positive. The diabetic Psammomys rats experienced reduced blood glucose levels. Some achieved normal levels. These levels were considered normal because they matched the levels of the animals in the controlled group that were not diabetic. There were also reduced plasma insulin, plasma cholesterol, and plasma triglyceride levels.

These normal animals also underwent the dietary program with no adverse effects. They experienced little reduction in glucose levels and no reduction in insulin levels. They also experienced reduction in cholesterol levels, which improved their health.

Overall, the diseased animals were healed, while the non-diseased animals were sustained. This makes good sense, for if good health can be re-acquired through a certain diet, it can be sustained by the same diet. This proves that this particular diet is not only beneficial for the person suffering a disease, but also for the disease-free person, as well.

These facets serve as points of interest when considering the possible and highly probable benefits of maintaining this type of diet for extremely longer periods, including a lifetime. Because of this, some people believe that human studies about the role of dietary restriction in disease prevention and tissue regeneration should be conducted with the Followers of the Honorable Elijah Muhammad. We have many accounts of the effectiveness of such a diet in curing diseases and in maintaining and sustaining life.

The most important findings from dietary restriction research were: 1) that all creatures studied, which includes cows, fruit flies, mosquitoes, and mice have achieved health benefits; and 2) all creatures studied demonstrated that long-term dietary restriction continued to improve the health of the creature. Researchers further agree that *life extension* is a by-product of a dietary regimen that lessens the disease. So is weight loss.

This fortifies the point previously made, which is that "weight loss" should not be the ultimate goal of obesity treatment. Life extension, as the ultimate aim, encompasses not only weight loss but also reductions in chronic disease risks.

On this note, we also revisit the "adding to" of Almighty God's divine dietary advice by the *merchants of death* and would-be scientists. As previously stated, the Honorable Elijah Muhammad mandates that adult humans eat only one meal a day, with no snacks between meals. At a minimum, we are to eat this one meal within a timeframe of several hours, and not eat again until the same time the next day.

Dietary restriction that merely limits the amount of food that a person eats at the same numerous meal settings is futile. For example, some nutritionists recommend eating three "small" meals, as a means of achieving weight loss. Yet, this will not achieve good health.

What difference does it make if a person reduces his or her food intake to only one plate of food at the five daily eating sessions, rather than the two plates usually consumed at each session? The digestive system is still in constant action, even though it is dealing with less food. Does this help the digestive process? NO! The digestive process is engaged whether we eat one cookie or a whole chicken.

In constantly eating, not only is the digestive organs kept consistently and completely involved in all phases of the digestive process, but also, the person risk not being able to properly digest any of the food eaten. We put ourselves into overload, which wears down our delicate digestive organs. This renders them ineffective in digesting food and, as a result, they degenerate and we become malnourished and diseased.

In fact, the entire body degenerates due to an over abundance of poison, and lack of vital nutrients. To further drive this point home, we consider the effects of overwhelming the pancreas, one of the body's most vital organs.

Pancreas Ambush

As previously discussed in Chapter 3, the pancreas is a very important organ because it produces the enzymes and hormones that aid the digestive process. As noted, all food components (not just starch) are responsible for pounding the pancreas, thereby injuring it. Of course, this is only when food is eaten more than once a day. Atrophy of the pancreas is the result of overeating.

In the book, *Amino Acids in Therapy*, Dr. Leon Chaitow explains the adverse health affects associated with pancreas malfunction. He writes:

> *A variety of factors can mitigate against the long-term pancreatic efficiency. These include the assault on it by the monumental amounts of sugar that it is obliged to handle via its insulin production...The first effects of such a pancreatic insufficiency are a reduction in bicarbonate production, leading to symptoms that are frequently dismissed as gastritis. Reduced enzyme activity and finally aberrant insulin production follow this.*

The last statement is another way of describing the condition of diabetes mellitus. The increase in sugar consumption that was previously addressed is a central cause of pancreas malfunction. So, after taking a constant pounding, the pancreas has difficulty producing the necessary substances to aid the digestive process. As it weakens, it produces less and less of the required digestive juices, and eventually fails. Let us read further. Dr. Chaitow states:

> *Inactivation of, or insufficiency in the production of, proteolytic enzymes from the pancreas...can result in poor digestion of amino acids. A further likelihood is that protein molecules might be absorbed in their undigested forms, which can provoke inflammatory reactions, sometimes in distant tissues and organs. If at the same time the circulating anti- inflammatory enzymes are deficient, as a further consequence of pancreatic exhaustion, then the ability of the body to deal with such inflammatory reactions (allergic or otherwise) will be reduced or absent.*

These adverse health conditions are arthritis and immunodeficiency diseases. It is safe to say that many people have not realized that arthritis is rooted in diet, and is associated with pancreas malfunction.

Some medical journals suggest that arthritis is related to the body's immune system. It develops when the body is unable to produce enough antibodies to prevent viruses from entering the joints.[162] This is true, however, amino acids are the primary building components of antibodies, so when they are deficient, antibodies are not produced. In some instances, antibodies are altered and unable to differentiate between viruses and healthy cells. Consequently, the antibodies destroy both.

Other medical scientists suggest that arthritis is produced from the absorption of undigested nutrients that permeate the intestinal lining causing inflammation in the joints. This also has merit. A weak stomach or small intestine cannot keep antigens and other harmful agents from entering the blood stream.

In either case, the depletion of pancreatic juices via the over consumption of food is central to these conditions. We continue:

> *The ability of pancreatic insufficiency to interfere with amino acid digestion is, however, our main concern. Should inadequate breakdown of ingested proteins take place, and amino acid deficiency result, despite high levels of first class protein in the diet, the consequences*

could include difficulty, or inability, on the part of the body to produce adequate enzymes, hormones, antibodies, and new tissue.

The likelihood would then also exist for excessive demands on a wide range of minerals and vitamins...leading to deficiencies in these. The immune system's ability to adequately defend the body under these conditions would be severely compromised.

Enzymes, hormones, and antibodies, as well as all body cells depend on protein to function properly. Without protein, the body degenerates, which is seen and identified as various diseases.

In pancreatic malfunction, not only is the body undergoing internal destruction, but external forces such as parasites, viruses, and bacteria are able to wage an assault and cause further damage, due to the collapse of the body's immune system. Logically, something that is drastically in self-decline cannot defend itself against intruders.

Unfortunately, nearly all people suffer and die from pancreas malfunction, as this debilitating scenario, described above, are played out day-in and day-out in the bodies of those persons making up both the overweight and non-overweight populations. This equates to billions of people. Included in this gigantic number are the scientists, doctors, pharmacists, engineers, politicians, and bankers who work in concert to transform the most absurd theories about health into death-dealing policies and products.

The frequency in which we eat is equally as, if not more, important than the types of foods eaten, especially when all foods contain some measure of poison. Of course, this does not mean that we should eat bad foods. It means that even good foods are harmful when eaten three and five times a day. This goes for vegetables, fruits, and grains. These are good foods but when the pancreas and other digestive organs are unable to manage these foods, they give the body little benefit, while causing further damage.

Consider This

Let us agree that eating one meal every 24 hours, at minimum, is the most logical and natural method of eating. Eating this way is in keeping with the mathematical operation of the human body, and as such, our lives are preserved when we follow the laws that govern life.

CHAPTER 7

Lifestyle Prescription

In the book, *FAQs About How To Eat To Live* (Vol. 1), I state:

A dietary prescription must identify the foods to eat, how these foods should be prepared, and the best time to eat these foods. These core factors support longevity, but only when such a prescription is based on science, specifically those sciences that relate to the human body, with emphasis on the digestion process... Therefore, an adequate dietary prescription must be in harmony with these biological and metabolic processes.

We have already established the best meal-time frequency, which is every 24 hours. The other essentials of this prescription are contained in the books *How To Eat To Live (Book 1 & 2)*; *FAQs About How To Eat To Live (Vols. 1& 2)*; *Nuts Are Not Good for Humans; and Whose Protein.*

In this chapter, we identify additional aspects that fortify the divine dietary prescription. These aspects are cautionary points, with respect to avoiding the various machinations of the merchants of death; and lifestyle recommendations that can aid our quest to obtain better health.

Weight Chart & Scales

Rarely has the subject of weight charts been mentioned in the many epidemiological and solution-oriented discussions about obesity. Nevertheless, there is a history to the use of weight charts and scales. We covered this point earlier. According to the back cover of *How To Eat To Live*, the dietary recommendations and weight charts published in 1959 by *U.S. News and World Report* were nearly verbatim to the papers the federal government took from the Honorable Elijah Muhammad in 1942 when they falsely arrested him.

This confiscated information included the dietary and health guidance the Honorable Elijah Muhammad received from Almighty God in the 1930s. Although, no epidemiological studies were conducted with His Followers during that time, we do know that they lived longer and maintained greater health than did the common people — those who ate many meals a day.

We also know that it was during the 1930s that studies into dietary or caloric restriction intensified. Little is known about what prompted these studies, but many believe that the dietary guidance taught by the Honorable Elijah Muhammad gave rise to this world's interest in this area. Despite this interest, this new dietary paradigm remains unknown to the general population.

Weight charts show height-to-weight relationships, and thus, provide "average" or "ideal" weight parameters. For example, a man or woman having a certain height should weigh a certain amount, or have his or her weight within a specific range. This "ideal" weight is healthy weight or weight that prevents weight-induced sickness and disease, which occurs through overweight or underweight.

The Honorable Elijah Muhammad used weight charts for several reasons. One reason was to empower His Followers to adequately assess their weight, and subsequently, make the proper adjustments to return to those "ideal" parameters — that is, if they happened to be beyond those parameters. Such adjustments could be achieved through various ways — fasting, eliminating certain foods from one's diet, reducing meal portions, or increasing exercise.

Tables 6 and 7 show the recommended average weights for men and women, respectively, that were published in the *1959 U.S. News and World Report* article.[163] Appendix C contains weight charts used by private and public institutions.

Weight charts and weight scales are tools that allow us to arrive at the facts, eliminating one's mystery about how much one might weigh. Additionally, these tools prevent us from signing on to the notion that we must look fat to be overweight. This is not so. As the cliché goes — "looks are deceiving".

The Honorable Elijah Muhammad's teacher, Master Fard Muhammad, required of Muslim women that they not be found weighing other than themselves. This also applies to all His

Followers, but the woman is emphasized for various reasons. How would they know what they should weigh without weight charts, and how would they learn their actual weight without stepping on a scale? Weight checks are conducted periodically, sometimes several times a week.

Anyone can get used to getting fat, especially considering that 20 or 30 pounds do not instantly jump on a person. Because weight is gradually gained, we are prone to deceive ourselves, until we are shocked into reality.

This reality check usually occurs when we are diagnosed with some weight-related chronic disease. Sometimes, even having to buy larger clothing is not enough to move people to consider their overweight condition and begin addressing it. Unfortunately, sickness and disease are the only motivators for many people.

Table 6: Weight Chart: Men

Height is with shoes on, weight is with ordinary indoor clothing				
Height	Age 30-39	Age 40-49	Age 50-59	Age 60-69
5' 2"	137	140	142	139
5' 4"	145	148	149	146
5' 6"	153	156	157	154
5' 8"	161	165	166	163
5' 10"	170	174	175	173
6' 0"	179	183	185	183
6' 2"	188	192	194	193
6' 4"	199	203	205	204

Table 7: Weight Chart: Women

Height is with shoes on, weight is with ordinary indoor clothing				
Height	Age 30-39	Age 40-49	Age 50-59	Age 60-69
5' 0"	120	127	130	131
5' 2"	126	133	136	137
5' 4"	132	140	144	145
5' 6"	139	147	152	153
5' 8"	146	155	160	161
5' 10"	154	164	169	*
* Average omitted because of lack of sufficient cases.				

By using weight charts and scales, a person can immediately learn if he or she has put on additional weight. The act of weighing one's self is a preventive measure. Why must a person wait until he or she looks fat or until disease sets in before deciding to learn of their weight? Is it not better to learn that you have picked up five pounds, and work to take off those pounds, then it is to watch the weight mount until such time that you feel shamed enough to confront the fact that you might have gained 20 or 30 extra pounds?

Such a revelation is not only demoralizing, but it also opens up a path to denial. A person wrestling with that amount of poundage might never get on a scale. For some, no news is good news, but this disposition is dangerous. In denying this weight gain, the person is opting to suffer and die.

Figure 19. Scale

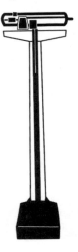

Additionally, being 20 or 30 pounds overweight sends that person "out of the gate" having an uphill climb to achieve proper weight. That person now must work exceedingly hard to come back in line with his or her ideal weight.

What also makes the road of having to drop 20 to 30 pounds an uphill battle is that the body has made adjustments to accommodate the excess fat. The potential to carry excess weight has been expanded. This is among the reasons why those who have crossed certain weight thresholds are always prone to regain the weight with ease. They have grown accustomed to carrying the excessive weight, so regaining it is not as traumatic as it was when the expansion first took place.

So knowing that 20 to 30 pounds must be taken off means that major efforts, rather than the minor ones, must be employed to get the weight within safe parameters. "Major" in this context means the journey is much longer than it would have been if only three or five pounds had to be lost.

This does not mean that a person should jump into a whimsical quick-fix weight-loss program, as an effort to get the weight off fast. As already stated, people must eat in accordance with the proper diet for humans — one-meal-a-day. Although this is a long process, it improves health, while safely reducing weight.

Again, if the person had been more aware of their weight through regular weight checks, the added weight would have been noticed, requiring a less burdensome effort. Obviously, having to knock off the three, four, or five pounds is much easier than having to drop 30 pounds.

Revisiting the back cover of *How To Eat To Live,* it states:

"He has cautioned his followers to be conscious of weight. Penalties are exacted from Muslim's found overweight."

With respect to the penalties exacted for carrying excess weight, we can surmise that the logic was and remains: "its better to pay now then to pay later." Good health is required of any people or nation, and such cannot be taken for granted, nor can such be treated in a trifling manner. If the goal of a nation is to advance with each generation, and all resources must be marshaled to ensure this advancement, then neither human nor financial resources can be lost due to ill-health, especially from poor eating habits.

Therefore, in the Nation of Islam, overweight was neither accepted nor tolerated. Those found overweight were reprimanded for their negligence and encouraged to address the condition.

As you know, our weight is usually taken when we visit the doctor. This is part of a medical pre-assessment routine, regardless of the nature of the visit (health checkup, sickness, etc.). Unfortunately, many people, especially poor people, are negligent about getting periodic checkups. Having no health insurance is often the excuse used to justify not getting routine health checks. Yet, people have the money to buy liquor, fast foods, and to "party". Health physicals are often less than $60.

Some people go years, even decades, without visiting a doctor. This is among the reasons why people learn that they have a disease when the disease is in its most progressive stage. This is usually the late stage. At this point, treatment options are few, and the prognosis for recovery is slim to none.

Periodic doctor visits still fall short when it comes to being mindful of our weight. Learning of our weight only when we visit the doctor, which is perhaps three or four times a year, is too infrequent. We must be constantly aware of our weight. Therefore, we should weigh ourselves, at least, once a week.

Discipline & Will Power

Lifestyle changes, as with any change, cannot occur unless the person has reached a level of dissatisfaction. The degree of dissatisfaction must be intense enough to propel the person to change. Just mild dissatisfaction on a *sometimey* basis will not do.

The Honorable Elijah Muhammad taught that 100% dissatisfaction brings about a total change. Less than 100% dissatisfaction might bring about moderate changes or no change. The latter is what takes place most of the time, because people usually vent dissatisfaction through their mouths, but do nothing to make conditions better.

This is because change requires effort. It requires concentration. It requires both mental and physical work. No significant changes can take place without discipline. Laziness and mindlessness are incompatible with change.

Anything that must be regulated is regulated through discipline. In this context, discipline is restraint against doing something contrary to that, which produces the better outcome. Discipline is achieved through knowledge and willpower.

To the injury of the obese person, scientists publicly question whether willpower actually exists. Additionally, many weight-loss researchers seem to think willpower is an outdated and discredited concept.[164] This disposition is a drastic change from the early 1950's, when willpower was deemed the most accepted concept in preventing obesity. People were encouraged to push away from the dinner table. Many things were quite simple during that era.

Now, the concept of "willpower" is considered outdated because of the awareness of the biological drivers of appetite, and an environment that makes food available at every turn — literally. Such a position is bogus and has only exacerbated the obesity pandemic. It has promoted weakness. It has obese people blaming everything except themselves, while they rest in comfort zones, digging their graves with their teeth.

Not only has the obese person developed a comfort zone, but those around them — his or her family members and friends, also adapt to seeing that person overweight. Over time, little is mentioned about their condition. Little is also done about it. We just get used to seeing them fat, just as they get used to being fat.

Also, over time, the feeling of shame is replaced by foolish defense mechanisms, as people vehemently defend their fatness. These defense mechanisms often ride on self-righteous posturing, complete with silly clichés, such as "love it or leave it", "love me as I am", "who said that I am overweight", or "I am comfortable with myself".

The travesty in this is that it goes against everything that makes us human. As Almighty God's greatest creation, there is nothing that humans cannot overcome. We have demonstrated this, individually and collectively. It is even demonstrated in the obesity pandemic.

For example, the awesome ability of humans to adapt to various physical conditions makes it easy for people to gain weight. Here, rest the problem. The reality is that people can easily get used to carrying excessive weight. They may never get physically comfortable being obese, but they have adapted mentally to seeing themselves overweight. Our adaptability puts us in comfort zones. Obesity is on the rise because many have developed comfort zones.

Even so, getting out of this zone follows a similar course — it is done gradually. It is done through a determined and made-up mind to stick to the proper diet for humans. As the saying goes — "there is nothing stronger than a *made up* mind. Too often, we get weak-minded in mid-stream, and then create false justifications to abort the struggle.

In this society, the pull of food is formidable, especially when food dens are everywhere and food commercials run rampant. This is the terrain. This is the world in which we live. Albeit, knowledge of this should empower us to stay the course.

With respect to knowledge, a person must know the dietary parameters on which discipline is applied. As for the health researcher who discredits willpower, one point must be established. That point is that without clearly delineating the precise diet that support health and longevity, who can be charged with the "lack of will-power". To boot, who can say that people lack willpower, especially when the diets they have been following promote obesity. It may be a matter of frustration rather than the lack of willpower.

Fortunately, we have established that *precise* diet on which obese people can mount and witness excellent results. This diet supports discipline because it is regulated.

Again, the Honorable Elijah Muhammad states that we must have regularity to everything. There is great wisdom in this. Discipline is inherent in a regulated or ordered life. After launching into this life, willpower becomes less and less a necessity, as we gradually live in the easy flow of a divine life.

Prepare Your Own Meals

To reiterate, societal conditions have most people, particularly parents, working longer hours under highly stressful conditions. People are rushed to complete nearly every human endeavor instantly, and this naturally cannot be done, so disease due to stress is rampant, communication is ineffective, and the much needed nurturing that each person requires is nearly nonexistent.

This era of "rush" has spilled over into our dietary habits. Time constraints have people eating snacks and meals in cars, on bikes, at bus stops, in restaurants, and at numerous places other than home. Nearly half the food ordered at fast food restaurants is now through the drive-up window. People's automobiles have become their dining rooms. This is among the greatest shifts in American society, and is a major contributor to obesity and diet-related diseases.

As acceptable as this bestial type of eating might be in America, in some places around the globe, this behavior is incomprehensible. For example, European nutritionists, visiting America, often remark that Americans are constantly chewing on the street, in museums, in church, and many other places. It seems as though Americans need to have something in their mouths at all times — cigarette, cigar, pipe, candy, gum, twig, lollypop, burger, French fry, potato chip, donut, etc. Just as babies, something must always be in their mouths to pacify their taste buds.

This unstable dietary practice is producing profound effects, which include chronic nutrient deficits of certain vitamins, minerals, and other food components. Medical researchers know that eating on the run is not conducive to proper digestion. In addition, ulcers and other digestive ailments result.

The hectic lifestyles of parents are being blamed for poor dietary habits across the board — of both children and parents. Again, the clearest evidence is the "family-gripped" obesity pandemic. There is a pool of research about childhood obesity. As previously noted, this is also pandemic. However, little research has focused on parenting as a central cause of obesity and other dietary-related diseases.

According to market research, children between the ages of five and nine years suffer from a negative *spillover effect* from parental lifestyles.[165] The researchers state:

> *There are numerous factors contributing to this worrying phenomenon, ranging from children's increasingly sedentary lifestyles, the Americanisation of...diet, and a decline in family meal occasions.*

This travesty has translated into the expansion of and increased sales of ready-made meals and snacks composed of chemical additives. These items have taken over the space in the refrigerator and cupboards. Again, Americans and persons living in industrialized countries spend nearly half of their food dollars on foods prepared away from home.[85] Unhealthy chemical-laden foods have been chosen at the expense of preparing more time-consuming, nutritious meals.

This *snowball* effect means that the sense of family has dissipated to nothingness. Longer working hours, an increase in the number of working women, and a need for exhausted parents to get a much-needed breather, have made the "family eating together" concept a thing of the past. Clearly, the old American traditions were better serving than the new behaviors. The researchers continue:

> *The fragmentation of family eating has resulted in a significant growth in 'child only meals' where child-specific foods or child-specific preferences such as chips and pizza are predominant.*

We already noted that children are targets of marketing frenzies by the *merchants of death*. Parents not only feed into this, but they support this nonsense wholeheartedly by purchasing these items. At what point did children need their unique "lot" of foods — specifically designed for them? And, what can these so-called foods be except microwavable, chemical-laden materials, deceptively called food?

Also, the bedroom culture has taken shape, as children are increasingly spending more time in their bedrooms becoming media junkies — watching sexually explicit, violent, and fantasy-ridden television programs, which advertise snacks by the minute. This is an aggressive and drastic form of brain-dirtying and manipulation. Antisocial, violent, dumbfounded, and zombie-like behaviors are the result. Some parents get more animated responses from turtles than from their children.

Many parents are at a loss of what to do with their children. The answer is quite simple: start acting like parents — teaching, training, counseling, and caring for your children. In the end, most parents will find themselves wishing that they had spent more time with their children. However, the clock can never be turned back, so it is best to make the proper adjustments now.

Throughout *How To Eat To Live*, the Honorable Elijah Muhammad constantly encourages us to prepare our meals. He also warns us of the consequences for not doing such. First, we must establish what "preparing" means. With the information presented thus far, we know that "preparing" does not mean putting a chemical-infested TV dinner in the oven or microwave. Nor does it mean putting condiments on fast foods (hamburgers, French fries, cheese steaks, hoagies, etc.).

There are many benefits to cooking our food — some obvious and some not so obvious. An obvious benefit is that preparing our own food ensures that it is not contaminated through the hands of others, especially in restaurants or the like. The less obvious is that we can gain *that* essential and vital sense of family many people so disparately need. This, alone, will not only eliminate adverse health risks, but also it will alleviate the mental and emotional plight experienced by parents and children by bringing about a sense of family.

Avoiding Foods

Certain types of foods must be totally avoided if good health is our objective. We cannot eat anything and everything, and expect to live a long and healthy life. This is a logical deduction. However, as logical as it may be, many people eat anything.

In the books, *How To Eat To Live*, the Honorable Elijah Muhammad brings to the forefront the subject of food distinctions — that is, food fit for humans, as opposed to foods fit for other creatures of the earth. There should be no doubt that certain animals prefer foods that humans cannot eat. There also should be no doubt that the digestive system in the human is different from those of other creatures, and that this uniqueness also determines the foods that it is made to digest. The simple solution is for us to eat human food and not animal food.

This animal food is pointed out in the books, *How To Eat To Live*. The scientific research that makes these foods fit for animals and not humans is contained in the books, *FAQs About How To Eat To Live* (Vols. 1 & 2), *Nuts Are Not Good for Humans*, and *Whose Protein* — by this author.

Fast Food

Fast food is highest on the list of foods to avoid. As noted throughout this book, part of the problem with obesity is that fast food death-dens are everywhere, affording everyone the opportunity to grab a burger, fries, shake, or other chemical-laden items. Fast foods have been linked to the obesity and chronic disease epidemics.[166]

The energy density of foods is a key determinant of energy intake, and fast foods are very dense foods. Fast foods have high fat and high sugar contents. Many studies that have assessed the composition of fast foods proved that most fast foods have an extremely high energy density.

At some fast food *joints*, the average energy density of the entire menu is very high. In fact, fast foods are 65% higher in energy than the average British diet and 145% higher than traditional African diets. High energy-dense snacks and fast foods currently contribute 11% of total dietary fat in the American diet.

The chemical construction of fast foods is also death-dealing, as this food promotes palatability but not satiety. Palatability is the pleasantness of food. It is related to the intake response towards a food. When you enjoy the taste, smell, and overall pleasantness of a food, you tend to eat more of that food. Fast food taste good, so people eat them often.

Satiety is the condition of being full or gratified beyond the point of satisfaction. It is the feeling we get after eating a good, wholesome and nutritious meal. After such a meal, the thought of returning to the table a few hours later for another serving does not come to mind. We have been well fed. This is not so with fast foods.

Although, high energy-dense foods are more palatable than low energy-dense foods, such as fruits and vegetables, low energy-dense foods promote satiety. Fast foods, not inducing satiation, cause a *'passive over-consumption'* of these foods. Most of us have experienced this. After eating fast foods, hunger seems to appear a few hours, if not moments, later — in spite of the super-sized entrée we already gobbled down.

Both short-term and long-term studies have demonstrated that fast foods, being high in fat and sugar disturb satiation[167] by challenging appetite control systems. Again, these biological systems are purposely manipulated through poisons placed in the foods. This is why fast food is a billion-dollar industry.[99]

Studies reveal that obese persons prefer dense foods, which are the very foods that cause weight gain and over consumption. Fast foods must be avoided.

No Seafood

In Chapter 3, we discussed how the synthetic chemical, *organochlorine*, is a major source of environmental contamination. These made-man poisons, although now banned from use, are linked to the obesity and diabetes epidemics. They negatively affect the body's (our bodies') neuroendocrine functions.

Surveys conducted in a number of countries have shown that the principal source of human exposure to organochlorines is through diet.[168] Therefore, avoiding these chemicals is not a legislative act of Congress, but our awareness of these toxins and our desire to avoid consuming them through our diets.

Seafood and meat are the major dietary sources of organochlorine contaminants. The lipophilicity of these toxins enables crustaceans, such as crabs, mussels, shellfish and other sea scavengers to absorb and harbor these chemicals in their flesh.

As you may know, Almighty God forbade the Children of Israel, and thus humanity, to eat these creatures. The essential reason, at that time, was and remains that these creatures are scavengers. Scavengers eat filth. Humans, as the Creator's greatest creation, are not designed to eat filth. Filth destroys us.

Today, this reason has been embellished by these creatures' ability to harbor chemical waste. When eating these foods, we are eating filth and toxins — both debilitating and deadly. And, because organochlorines pass higher up the marine life food chain to include fish, we are advised not to eat fish weighing more than

10 pounds. The larger the fish, the more of these toxins they have in their flesh.

Approximately 97% of the fish in the U.S. are contaminated by organochlorines.[169] This includes fish weighing less than 10 pounds. For this reason, health researchers recommend that people reduce their intake of organochlorine-contaminated fish. We may need to stop eating fish, altogether. Many people already do. In fact, Minister Louis Farrakhan has mandated members of the Nation of Islam to stop eating fish. This is wise guidance.

Simple Foods

This world promotes variety as a means of bringing excitement to life's most common activities. Eating is one of these activities. Therefore, most people in so-called industrialized countries have a long list of foods they eat. We can debate whether excitement is achieved through having radically different foods to eat each day. At a certain point, people will have to start creating not only dishes, but also foods. The chemical industry has done precisely this, creating chemical concocted foods that cater to those who must have something different to eat each day.

The Honorable Elijah Muhammad advised His followers to eat the simple foods. He positioned that we do not need a long list of foods to achieve good health. This makes sense and is irrefutable. After all, if the body can gain the nutrients it needs through one or two foods, the purpose of eating is achieved. One's taste buds may require variety, but the body is only interested in having what it needs to sustain itself. Also, simple foods taste good.

There is rich wisdom to this specific directive. For example, with variety comes the risk of consuming chemicals that impede nutrition. Ready-to-eat foods and so-called meal helpers are drenched with chemicals. Not only do these foods hinder digestion, but also they increase the risk of consuming hormone-mimicking poisons.

Additionally, the concept of variety is only a notion. According to an ERS report, variety is linked to poor food quality.[170] The report states:

The greater number and variety of food outlets do not offer any greater variety of basic foods, only more ways in which commodities can be formulated to foster the illusion of greater variety. Nor do the many outlets offer improved freshness or quality. On the contrary, the greater array of prepared foods offer less freshness, reduced nutrients, and higher costs than common basic foods freshly prepared in the home.

It comes down to the fact that chemicals cost money. It is less expensive to grow a vegetable than it is to process synthetic chemicals to make foods, or so-called foods. Is there such a thing as fresh chemicals? No. Therefore, if you want chemical-laden foods, then you will spend more money than necessary, while injuring your health.

The area of *food-to-food* interactions on digestion is gaining attention. People are realizing that certain foods do not mix well. With variety comes the risk of harmful food-to-food and nutrient-to-digestive enzyme interactions. People who consume huge meals comprised of meats, vegetables, processed foods, chemical-concocted foods, forbidden swine flesh, and other scavengers have transformed their stomachs into melting pots of disease and self-destruction.

The Honorable Elijah Muhammad's recommendation that we eat the bodacious navy bean, wheat bread, and whole milk ensures that no hormone-mimicking chemicals are consumed, and that food-to-food interactions promote health rather than destroy it.

All the while, the body is provided the nutrients required to sustain it. What better guidance is there?

Fasting

The Honorable Elijah Muhammad writes in *How To Eat To Live*:[171]

Fasting is a greater cure of our ills — both mentally and physically …We can take medicine all of our lives until it kills us, but we are still ailing with the same old diseases.

Most of us can attest to this. Again, medicine is a temporary relief, but is never a cure. Despite this, some physicians advise people to take medication for months, even years. Logically, why would anyone take a pill for one, two or three years? This does not make sense. The drug industry has influenced people to make medications a part of their diets.

They do this by painting digestive conditions as long-term bouts. They can then prescribe pills for a long time and make billions of dollars. For example, antiulcerants and cholesterol reducers were the top leading classes of drugs sold in 2001 and 2002.[172] Antiulcerants allegedly treat stomach ulcers. Sales of this nostrum totaled $21.9 billion last year. Cholesterol/triglyceride reducers raked in $21.7 billion in sales. The demand for Lipitor, a cholesterol treatment and the top-selling drug worldwide, had much to do with the growth of this class of nostrums.

People take these drugs daily for years. They believe that as long as they take the drug, they will become or stay healthy. This is far from the truth. For example, studies have determined that any alleged reduction in heart disease due to lipid-lowering drugs is offset by a rise in noncardiovascular mortality. Among this mortality were increases in suicide and violence due to mental illnesses.[173]

Consequently, anti-depressant drugs are ranked third in sales, at $17.1 billion a year, coming behind lipid reducers. So, it appears that people taking lipid-lowering drugs need anti-depressant drugs to keep from going insane.

And, as previously noted, drugs create other health ailments that lead to poor quality living and early mortality. This nonsense reflects the dietary dark ages, showing that nothing has changed.

We reiterate that drugs are not on record as having cured anyone of anything. This is not the case with fasting, as this modality has cured people of many ailments. Fasting is a dietary practice. It normalizes and balances the body fluids. It does this by allowing the body time to rest and cleanse itself.

Mentally, fasting strengthens our willpower. It helps us gain control over natural biological drives that, if uncontrolled, have the potential to destroy us. Appetite is one of the greatest drives, and as we see in obesity and chronic disease pandemics, this drive is causing anguish and misery. You will also find that fasting allows you to control the sexual drive. It also improves patience, thus lowering one's blood pressure.

The Honorable Elijah Muhammad mandates His Followers to fast as often as possible. For example, we are required to fast, at least, 3 days each month. I also know of people who fast one day each week.

Mastering one-meal-a-day is similar to fasting for one day — 24 hours. You can then increase your fast to two days and so forth.

Exercise

There is enough data to support that lower physical activity levels, the lack of exercise and a sedentary lifestyle are associated with adult and childhood obesity. This is also an easy deduction. We cannot just sit around day-in and day-out and not exercise. Exercise is essential in obtaining and enjoying a healthy life.[174] It has proven to help aid weight loss in obesity treatments[107] and to lower blood-sugar levels in diabetes patients.[175]

If we do not have the time to exercise, then we must carefully consider if we are justified in eating. One of the benefits of exercise is that we are able to burn off calories. We expend energy during exercise or during higher levels of physical activity, which requires us to replenish our bodies by eating food.

The Honorable Elijah Muhammad required His Followers to exercise daily. This could include brisk walking, jogging, weight training, or participating in recreational sports, such as volleyball, swimming, basketball, etc. Numerous activities can offer us a way of exercising. Eating one meal a day, combined with exercise, leads to optimal health.

Stress-Driven Obesity

The Honorable Minister Louis Farrakhan teaches that some stress is motivational. This type of stress is associated with our responsibilities. This is healthy stress, and is not meant to destroy us. However, when we are not upholding our responsibilities to Almighty God, to our families, to ourselves, and to our communities, this stress intensifies and can become injurious. As we fulfill our God-given obligations, this stress is manageable.

There is also unhealthy stress, which most of us experience at varying levels. This stress is associated with a world driven by profit, where anguish, disease and death are inborn. It is this rat-race society, wherein most people have to work themselves into the ground to eek out a living. Everything, including human rights, has a price tag attached to it. This has created unusual and unnecessary stress, producing the dog-eat-dog world in which we live.

Consequently, a person who has no money will be homeless, hungry and uneducated — a life on the verge of worthlessness, which brings extraordinary stress. And, in such a society, no person is exempt from demonic capitalistic factors that can potentially send him or her to the unemployment lines. As a result, each adult faces unnecessary stress levels.

It is no surprise that obesity is on the rise because there is comfort in food. Because most of us live under the constant burden of stress, the demand for comfort is extreme, so we become sex addicts, food addicts or drug addicts. Recent studies have confirmed that people eat comfort foods to relieve chronic stress, and consequently, get fat.

In some experiments, scientists have matched human behavior with that of rodents. Eating high fat and high sugar foods caused the rats to produce more of a stress hormone releaser in their brains.[176] It is no wonder why fast food chains are everywhere. They serve as instant, yet temporary, *fixes* to relieve stress.

Scientists have engaged human studies to examine the associations between stress-related eating and drinking, and obesity, as factors predicting this behavior. One study comprised 2,359 men and 2,791 women.[177] All of them were born in 1966.

The results indicated that the BMI of persons at 31 years of age was highest among stress-driven eaters and drinkers, especially women. Stress-driven eaters tended to eat more sausages, hamburgers, pizza, chocolate and other dense foods than other people do. Also, stress-driven eaters consumed more alcohol than other people did.

Even more interesting is that scientists learned that the best predictors of stress-related eating and drinking among men were: 1) being single or divorced, 2) a long history of unemployment, 3) an academic degree, and 4) a low level of occupational education. Among women, the best predictor was a lack of emotional support.

Researchers concluded that programs aimed at preventing and treating obesity should cover the way in which people deal with emotions, ways of achieving greater emotional support, and strategies for handling stress caused by unemployment or work.

In an insightful article published in Essence Magazine, overweight Black women — from a wide cadre of social and professional backgrounds — shared similar themes as the reasons for their exccessive weight. Heartache, daily stress, childhood wounds, and job-related burnout were drivers for overeating.[178]

Animal stress research has revealed interesting insights. Studies in mouse 'societies' identified two principal types of stress reactions — one successful and one unsuccessful. After a period of strain, successful mice ended up in a superior position, with advantages for feeding, reproduction, etc. Also, the hormonal–autonomic consequences showed increased activity of the sympathetic nervous system and increased sex steroid levels.[179] The stress improved the mice.

The unsuccessful mice had defeat reactions. These mice were unable to cope with a competitive situation and developed a reaction characterized by submissive behavior and helplessness, and were socially handicapped. Their hormonal reaction was dominated by decreased secretions of sex steroid hormones.

Similar experiments have been performed in non-human primates, with essentially the same results. The animals with a defeat type of reaction accumulated excess fat in visceral adipose tissue and developed insulin resistance, dyslipidaemia, hypertension, impaired glucose tolerance and early signs of coronary atherosclerosis. They simply could not adapt to the competitive environment so they died a slow and painful death. These experiments are eye-openers for us.

There is little doubt that the world in which we live is not only competitive, but also inhumane and wicked. Consequently, scores of lives are destroyed as many find it difficult to cope. Addictions are high, and disease runs rampant. Fortunately, divine guidance comes to help us cope and succeed. This leads to the next aspect of this lifestyle prescription.

Spiritual Perception

In the Bible, the dietary dark ages is characterized as a world of sin. We are born into this world and shaped by the dominant societal conditions, which spring from the mind of the *merchants of death*, the *comfortable beneficiaries* or *Satan*. These conditions are iniquitous, and they frame our behaviors and lifestyles. The result is death because the lifestyle practice is a death-style practice.

According to the Scriptures, those who desire to rise above the world of iniquity are required to not be "of this world", nor to love it.[180] They are mandated to "put on the whole amour of God that they may be able to stand against the wiles of the devil".[82] However, neither can be accomplished until the divine guidance capable of achieving such comes. This divine guidance includes spiritual awareness and practices that enable us to transcend the world of iniquity.

This guidance comes at the end of the rule of the wicked, which is now, and gives us the "lifestyle" of God. This Guidance is presented and made available to us through the Teachings of the Honorable Elijah Muhammad and Minister Louis Farrakhan. Through this Guidance, we also obtain rich spirituality — something impossible to gain under the rule of the wicked.

Generally, spirituality denotes a belief in a Being and/or an Existence higher than ourselves, and higher than the temporal plain that we encounter day-to-day. In spiritual development, we can obtain the power to transcend the stresses of life, because we are able to think beyond the "seen" and realize that we are blessed with this wondrous gift called life. It is through this appreciation that we find real comfort. No matter what happens to us, as Believers in the Almighty, we know that we remain blessed.

Appreciation and gratitude are intrinsic to spirituality, and when these attitudes are combined with compassion, then we are really in the realm of security and comfort. Compassion gives us a charitable spirit. We will lend a hand, volunteer to help another person, coach and teach children in athletics, music, etc., or counsel the mentally ill.

In other words, the apex of spirituality is that we are driven by compassion to perform acts of kindness. This supports longevity by removing stress, because there is great consolation in making real changes in the lives of others. Much too often, we are focused on our own problems and pains. In many cases, the answer to solving our own problems rests in helping others. This leads to the final recommendation — change.

Making Changes

Of course, making lifestyle changes require fundamental adjustments in one's current view of life, as well as in one's life activities. We cannot do the same things and expect different outcomes. Therefore, we must arrange a schedule that allows us time to cater to our physical, intellectual and spiritual development. We have to set goals in these areas.

Goal-setting for personal development is often the first casualty in a societal climate dominated by greed. People easily set goals for things that make them more marketable — completing college, taking a course, etc. No doubt, these are important. Meanwhile, moral and spiritual goals are neglected, and these become the very things that derail people from other pursuits. So, lawyers, doctors, and engineers are steeped in substance abuse and other forms of self-destruction. Why? Money does not bring true satisfaction. Spiritual and moral development does.

We have learned that the only thing *constant* is *change*. Everything changes, including us — at least, physically. We get older and our bodies show it. However, certain mental habits or dispositions become too concrete in our lives. These also need to change. Some need to be thrown out of our minds.

There is no doubt that certain bad, unhealthy or unproductive habits are associated with a climate that breeds obesity and poor health. Adjustments to or elimination of these activities produces change, thus enabling us to adopt new habits that work in concert with our goals of acquiring and maintaining good health.

For example, a sedentary lifestyle is usually associated with eating in the bedroom, on the sofa, or in an extremely relaxing position. Soon after we eat that meal or snack, many of us simply fall to sleep. The consequence is weight gain and lethargy.

Simple adjustments, such as eating at the dinner table, produce radical changes in one's health and weight. Even more, people can determine that they will confine their meals to the dinner table, thus opting not to take the dessert to the bedroom or den, too.

Additionally, many people sit through hours of TV programs without doing any form of exercise when they can easily watch television while exercising. This simple adjustment can produce great benefits. We must discard those habits that impede our lives.

Obesity Drugs: A Deadly Hoax

The following is from Chapter 5 of the first edition of *Obesity, Diabetes & How To Eat To Live*.

Some government officials agree that diet has the central role in staving off weight and disease. The August 16-18,1996 issue of USA WEEKEND, featured (former) FDA chief David Kessler. He is reported as saying, *"It really is changing your diet. The only answer is to stop eating a lot"*, when commenting on his 55 pound drugless weight-loss.

Despite this truth, the FDA, while under his watch, approved its first diet pill in 23 years, Redux. The sales of this drug *"are expected to reach $600 million a year"*. They were sure to mention this motive in the article. This is probably why a great deal of controversy surrounds the diet pill. The article addresses this controversy, so let's briefly deal with a few of these points.

As early as February 1995, the FDA refused to approve the obesity drug, *"partly because of the manufacturer's inadequate look at the potential for human brain damage."* Six prominent brain scientists warned the FDA that the results of the animal experiments with the drug caused brain damage from dosages that would be similar to those prescribed to patients. The article states:

> *The negative decision was made after a day of debate between company scientists who held that dexfenfluramine was not 'neurotoxic' and concerned researchers who called for human trials. Also fear was heightened at that time by a recent European finding that dexfenfluramine increased the odds of contracting a rare lethal heart-lung disorder.*

At the close of the meeting, FDA drug evaluator director, James Bilstad, suggested that another meeting be held with panel members to discuss the issues of risks verses benefits. He wanted to know if they would approve Redux if they weighed its risks and benefits rather than the safety of the drug. What kind of logic is this to base a decision? Who's side was he on, anyway? As a member of the FDA, you would think that he would have terminated the discussion until studies were made that concluded that neither brain damage nor the rare and lethal heart-lung disorder was associated with the drug. What benefits of the drug can possibly outweigh these death-dealing risks?

Following is the outright evil work of the *merchants of death*. The article goes on to state:

> *None of the outside scientists who opposed Redux because of the brain damage question attended that November 16 meeting. All of them already had planned to be in San Diego for the annual Society of Neuroscience convention. In early October, two of those scientists, professors Mark Molliver and Lewis Seiden of John Hopkins and Chicago Universities, wrote to committee members to make sure they received proper background literature. They also protested the hearing date, to no avail.*

Bilstad stood on the grounds that those scientists were invited and refused to come, but Mr. Seiden said that this was not true. He insisted that he wasn't officially invited. Mr. Molliver said the FDA informed him that the meeting was going to be held on November 17, but uninvited him a week before the meeting was held. This is pathetic, in the truest sense of the word. This is your FDA -the one that protects you and me.

So, when the Honorable Louis Farrakhan implicates the government as part of this death-dealing quartet, don't look at him as if he's paranoid. He isn't. Why should he be? He's living according to the Teachings of the Honorable Elijah Muhammad, which has his cabinets empty of medications, while the majority of the people continue to be victimized (through false advice and poison drugs) by the wicked. It's the ignorant masses that he's trying to save — who take every word coming from Satan (government) as gospel. Let's go further.

During the second meeting, the panel members were instructed to weigh the drug's risks verses benefits. So, after the manufacturers of Redux cowardly attacked the brain damage data in the absence of the original opposing scientists, the drug was approved by a 6-5 vote. The article states:

On Dec. 7, twenty-two brain scientists urged the FDA to 'forgo the final decision' until more information is available on potential brain damage in humans. Says Kessler: 'Don't believe for a moment that this drug is without risks. The question before the agency was: Would a rational person in consultation with a rational physician want to take this drug?'

I argue that the real question before the agency was, "How can we covertly appease the powerful drug industry?" Through lying, conniving and pulling several whammies, they got the job done. Concerning Mr. Kessler's weak response to the decision, I ask, "What makes a person rational? "A better question is, "What is the basis for rational thinking? "It's truthful information. So, does that mean that this article or a similar document (bearing the events by which Redux was approved) is going to be wrapped around the pill bottle? Hell no! The drug is painted as salvation for the obese.

The last sentence of the article states:

Marketer Wyeth-Ayerst says Redux, with diet and exercise, is an effective treatment for obesity, a chronic disease that contributes to 300,000 deaths each year.

The wicked nerve to include exercise and diet with this toxic drug! They used the phrase 'effective treatment', as a means of justifying this death-inducing diet pill. The USA TODAY article didn't take us back to 1994, when the drug was knocked down by scientists from Johns Hopkins Medical Institution. They confirmed that this drug, dexfenfluramine, caused extensive brain damage in monkeys tested over a one and half year period. Their summary sent Interneuron Pharmaceuticals' stock tumbling.

Now, the company's stock has risen considerably since the approval. It went from $6 to over $39 a share in less than two years. Investors were waiting for the drug's approval and leaped to fuel the company with money when it was approved. The FDA ignored bundles of evidence to appease these sick demons. Now, this drug is going to hurt and maim folks, while the stockholders get paid-in-full. How can I state this so confidently?

Well, dexfenfluramine is a drug that has been proven effective in obese animals because it increases the neurotransmitter, serotonin, which has been found to quail appetite. Sounds like the same story the other fellows told about the hormone, leptin. These mad scientists believe that increasing serotonin levels will halt the signals that make the body call for food. Again, is the biological signal the problem, or are "the eyes bigger than the stomach", when considering the cause of obesity?

It just so happens that other scientists have connected serotonin, to pain, sleep, anxiety, and depressive disorders. The scientists who are involved in the study of sleeping disorders tout increased serotonin levels as a means of inducing sleep, while other scientists seek increased serotonin levels for depressive disorders. So, when a person takes the diet pill for obesity, what other effects await him or her? Many! According to all the above, that person will not be depressed, anxious, or hungry, but sleepy. The truth is that he or she will be spaced-out. Did they tell the people that a side effect of this diet pill is withdrawal, or did folks not know that this is a "get-high" drug?

That's exactly what it is, and scientists fear that it will post the same adverse effects as amphetamines did in the 50s and 60s when they were used for obesity treatments. Now, they are regarded as controlled substances, along with cocaine, crack, and other behavioral altering drugs.

When you consider the role that serotonin has in treating hallucinations, drug abuse, cardiovascular disease, and migraines, it is evident that many hands are on this neurotransmitter. In fact, too many hands are on this substance. Multitudes of quacks are claiming some benefit from the inducement of serotonin levels. One wonders if each scientist knows what the other scientists are doing. The smell of disaster is quite apparent. Yet, in all these purported uses, the actual neuronal mechanisms and pathways producing these alleged therapeutic benefits have not been established.

The following comes from the *Encyclopedia of Human Biology*:

Brain serotonergic neurons have been demonstrated to mediate, in part, the hypothalamic regulation food intake. Drugs that act either directly or indirectly to increase 5-HT stimulation decrease food intake in rats. Such drugs include serotonin-releasing drugs such as P-chloroamphetamine and fenfluramine, which have been marketed as anti-obesity drugs in the clinical setting.

In addition, the selective 5-HT uptake inhibitors fluoxetine and zimelidine have been demonstrated to decrease body weight in non-depressed obese patients. Conversely, several direct acting 5-HT agonists, including 8-OH-DPAT, busipirone, and ipsoirone, have recently been reported to increase food intake in rats. Clearly, serotonin has a role in mediating the responses associated with food intake; however, the neuronal circuitry and receptors mediating the regulation of food intake remain unestablished.

Now we can understand why those 22 leading brain scientists were upset at the notorious and malicious acts of the FDA in approving a drug with extraordinary doubt attached to it. Again, it's all about money, and which drug company can best seize a vulnerable obese population.

Yet, if you read the articles about this new diet pill in periodicals other than those that are scientific, you would believe that this pill is the best thing going. This is because the same people that control the banks, drug industry, and government, control the media, too. It's all one big damnable hoax, and obese people are the targets.

Furthermore, studies conducted on Redux were very modest and fell substantially below standards in proving the drug's effectiveness. One article states the following:

> *First, the drug is not very effective, by the drug agency's (FDA) standards... The pill does not eliminate the need to diet, and the drug agency considers the difference of only six pounds after a year to be a marginal result. Because no studies have carried on beyond the year, it is not clear what happens after the patients come off the diet for long periods of time, or when they come off the drug...*

This gives us a behind-the-scenes look at the flaws in the studies that were conducted on the drug. It is obvious that more in-depth studies were warranted. Doesn't it seem reasonable to want to know the specifics about the effects that will result after a person decides to terminate use of a medication? Why approve a drug without this vital aspect of research? Let's read on:

> *A second issue is the drug's possible toxicity to brain cells. Redux works in the brain's limbic system by increasing the available amount of a substance called serotonin that helps transmit signals between brain cells. The drug prevents serotonin already working from being broken down and stimulates cells to produce more.*

> *Serotonin is a crucial factor in mood control in people. For example, the most effective and popular antidepressant drug, Prozac, also works to increase serotonin supplies by preventing serotonin from being broken down. And, because appetite control is linked to mental systems governing mood and stress, Prozac also has the side effect of reducing appetite in some patients being treated for depression.*

> *There is therefore a fear that Redux may cause problems in the same mood-regulating system. Dr. Lewis Seiden, a pharmacologist at the University of Chicago who was one of several critics who testified against the approval of the drug before the agency's advisory panel, said he and others had published studies of the drug or a closely related one*

in different animal species. He said they had shown that after taking the drug for some time and then stopping, the animals had severely depleted levels of serotonin.

In humans, that might be expected to produce a sudden severe depression or bursts of impulsive behavior, he said.

So, no one really knows what will happen when folks use the drug for long periods. Nor, do they know what will happen when they come off the drug -- if they can ever stop using it. One would not be off base to suggest that the drug's sales will continue to skyrocket as folks become "hooked." Maybe then, another drug will be developed to unhook them. Is this not Satan's program? Does not the treatment for persons addicted to drugs include the use of other drugs?

Interneuron Pharmaceuticals, Inc., stated that they would do post-marketing surveillance to keep an eye on this adverse effect in humans; however, what's that worth? Once drugs are approved for marketing, it's hard to get them unapproved and seized from the shelves, especially when wealthy investors have an interest in the product. This drug will simply join the FDA's watch list along with the other death-inducing drugs. And, these vile demons have the nerve to have higher learning degrees and certificates plastered on their walls. They falsely claim themselves as scientists, doctors, and business managers when they're not much above the cave man standards of their savage ancestors.

The information given above should raise questions concerning the integrity of the FDA. It should also create great apprehension for obesity drugs. Outright poison has been approved for marketing. This seems almost unreal, but it happens to be very real.

Unfortunately, many people have decided to consume obesity drugs. Folks are lured by ads that boast that a person can quickly lose unwanted pounds without dieting. Taking these drugs will allow a person to have their cake and eat it, too — along with the toxic pills. The April 7, 1997 issue of Drug Topics states the following in a column entitled, *Fat's in the Fire*:

The stampede of overweight Americans to obesity drugs has jingled retail pharmacy's cash registers, but it's also set off alarm bells in some quarters about the long-term effects of such therapy.

According to the article, this past January saw 2.3 million prescriptions issued, generating $62 million in sales. Primary care physicians were the major writers of obesity drug prescriptions. They issued 71% of these death-dealing chemicals. The sad fact is that 78% of obesity drugs are paid out-of-pocket because most insurance companies do not cover them. Astonishingly, some doctors offer programs that cost over $1,000 for a six-month supply. This is completely ridiculous. The article continues:

> America's flaming passion for obesity drugs has some pharmacists worried. Critics of fen-phen and dexfenfluramine are concerned that the medications are being inappropriately prescribed for people who want to lose a few pounds before swimsuit season, not for the truly obese.

This 'worry' stems from the incidence of primary pulmonary hypertension (PPH). The condition is one of several side effects associated with appetite suppressant drugs. This side effect is the lethal heart-lung disorder that they ignored to approve the drug, Redux. For the sake of information, let us take a moment to explain PPH.

While the *merchants of death* declare that increasing the serotonin level fools the body into believing its full, the lungs become overwhelmed with the substance and a host of adverse conditions result. The following six points are from PharmInfoNet's online discussion of obesity drugs:

Response 1: Dexfenfluramine may cause primary pulmonary hypertension as follows (personal communication from Camilla Cracchiolol):

1. Serotonin binds to receptors in lung tissue and causes vasoconstriction.

2. Drugs that inhibit the clearance of serotonin from lung tissue prolong the vasoconstriction and this is what leads to the pulmonary hypertension, via destruction of alveolar tissue and small blood vessels from lack of oxygen. The destruction of lung tissue makes the lungs stiff and not very pliable. Deoxygenated blood is pumped into the lungs by the right side of the heart. The blood picks up oxygen and returns to the left side, to then be delivered to the rest of the body via the left ventricles. When the lungs are stiff, and the small blood vessels in the alveoli are constricted, the heart has to pump much harder to get the same amount of blood in. This is pulmonary hypertension, which you

can have completely independent of high blood pressure in the rest of the body. The pulmonary hypertension, in turn, is what causes the damage to the heart. If the heart can't generate enough pressure to get all the blood into the lungs, it backs up. Over time, this stretches the heart wall and can also cause great damage to the small valves in the right side of the heart. This is bad news.

3. Dexfenfluramine has a relatively strong effect on the clearance of serotonin from pulmonary tissues compared to other anorexants. Hence its vasoconstrictive effect is stronger than most other anorexants. The rate of pulmonary hypertension from dexfenfluramine appears to be about 1 case in 40,000.

4. Both phentermine and chlorphetermine are mentioned in several studies. Chloraphentermine appears to be a slightly different drug with a much higher rate of pulmonary hypertension than phentermine HC1. And, the chlorinated versions of anorexant drugs all appear to have much more effect on lung tissue than the non-chlorinated varieties.

5. Phentermine HC1 by itself does two things:

• It inhibits serotonin uptake by pulmonary tissues.

• However, it *also* inhibits serotonin clearance.

*There *are* reports of pulmonary hypertension in humans from phentermine alone, although it's much rarer than with fenfluramine. The only reports of pulmonary hypertension from phentermine alone that this search turned up were in animal models; however several of these abstracts mentioned human cases as having occurred as though it is a well established fact.*

1. It's conceivable that phentermine could have an ameliorating effect on fenfluramine risk, as Dr. Pietr Hitzig asserts, by lowering the rate of serotonin uptake in pulmonary tissues. However, theoretically the combination of phentermine and fenfluramine could also act synergistically and increase the risk of pulmonary hypertension in at least a few individuals due to the fact that both drugs slow the rate of serotonin clearance from the lungs. This would depend on whether the reduction in the rate of pulmonary serotonin uptake is less or more than the reduction in pulmonary serotonin clearance. This would be determined by quirks in individual body chemistry, like the amount and exact configuration of certain enzymes (which can vary slightly for genetic reasons), how much serotonin the person produces in the first place, etc.

When this condition, PPH, was determined, Wyeth-Ayerst revised Redux's label to reflect a higher risk than was originally reported. It is a common practice among drug companies to revise labels after folks have been injured from using their drugs. Since most clinical trials are extremely ineffective, the general populace becomes the true clinical trial after the drugs are approved for marketing. As demonstrated, this approval is usually done in vicious fashion with the acquisition of money as the objective, not the health of the people. So, when these adverse effects begin to surface, drug companies merely revise the label to include the condition. This is all they do. The drug remains on the market. One would think that if automobiles are recalled for dangerous flaws, why would not lethal drugs be pulled off the shelves?

Unfortunately, PPH is not the only side effect of Redux. Others include diarrhea, dry mouth, and somnolence. In addition, many physicians are waiting for other side effects to surface. The article, *Fat's In The Fire*, ends with these words:

> *Rosenberg agreed that nothing can be done to stem the rising tide of obesity drugs. "Medicine is a business, and this is a huge market," he commented 'It has sex appeal. People coming in want it. If one physically won't do it, the next one will have to wait for the adverse drug reactions and the lawsuits. There will be a payback at some point.*

Now this pleasure-seeking mentality has more than half of Black women overweight, making them the primary candidates for obesity drugs. In a forthcoming report, we will present historical legislation that prohibited research entities from using Black women as human subjects for medical studies. Yes, Black women were the primary subjects for research in the previous century. We can strongly argue that nothing has changed. This is no great revelation. There have been paybacks with most drugs. Most recently there was a payback with the Norplant, a contraceptive that was marketed by Wyeth-Ayerst, as well. The Honorable Louis Farrakhan did his best, via the Final Call and public addresses, to warn folks, particularly Black women, not to use this poison. However, many did use it to their detriment. The pursuit of pleasure without regard for responsibility has allowed the merchants of death to destroy us.

I had a conversation with a Black woman about the obesity drug, Redux. Ironically, she informed me that she had just started using the drug, unaware that I was researching and writing about this subject. She had received a six-week supply that cost her hundreds of dollars. Of course, I took the time to inform her about my research and that she should cease from using the drug. It was my responsibility to do so regardless of the advice from her physician. I gave her Almighty God's instructions for weight control in *How To Eat To Live*.

Weeks later I happened to meet her again. She admitted that she continued to use the drug for a few weeks despite what I had told her. She was frustrated by her weight and had already made the investment, so she decided to go on using the drug. However, she finally was forced to stop using Redux. She said that she began to have headaches and was becoming very forgetful. She constantly felt heavy-headed. When she remembered what I had told her, she knew that it was time to stop using the drug. I was happy for her.

I wonder how many Black women have been instructed to use this drug by their physicians, especially when their doctors can make a substantial profit by prescribing the drug? I would hope that How To Eat To Live can one day become the dietary law of Black people. Drugs should never be placed in our veins, especially not for the purpose of losing weight.

The Honorable Elijah Muhammad states in How To Eat To Live that drugs will kill us. He states that we should never use drugs to address ailments caused by improper eating habits.[181] We should be ashamed to do so. He advises us to submit to the instructions from Almighty God, Who Came in Person of Master Fard Muhammad, to save us. We would be very wise to accept this advice, especially when the other alternatives only lead to our destruction.

Current Diabetes Drugs

NOTE: This is only a partial list of the diabetes drugs currently available on the market. Other diabetes drugs not listed here include Avandamet (Avandia + metformin), Glucovance (glyburide/metformin) and Glycet.

Diabetes Nostrum	Claim	Risk Factors
Actos (pioglitizone)	Actos works by improving the body's response to its natural supply of insulin, rather than increasing its insulin output. Actos also reduces the production of unneeded sugar in the liver.	Headache, hypoglycemia, muscle aches, respiratory tract infection, sinus inflammation, sore throat, swelling, tooth disorder, Anemia, shortness of breath, weight gain.
Amaryl (glimepiride)	Amaryl helps your body produce extra insulin when it is needed (after meals), so it can carry glucose into your cells to be converted into energy. Amaryl may also make tissues in your muscles and other organs more sensitive to insulin.	Severely low blood-sugar levels, dizziness, weakness, headache, nausea, and liver and kidney aggravation.
Avandia	Avandia works to help overcome insulin resistance by making the body's cells more sensitive to insulin.	Upper respiratory tract infection, injury, headache, back pain, hyperglycemia, fatigue, sinusitis, diarrhea, hypoglycemia.
Glipizide (Sulfonlyurea)	Glucotrol controls diabetes by stimulating the pancreas to secrete more insulin. Occasionally, type 2 diabetics must take insulin injections on a temporary basis, especially during stressful periods or times of illness.	Constipation, diarrhea, dizziness, drowsiness, gas, headache, hives, itching, low blood sugar, nervousness, sensitivity to light, skin rash and eruptions, stomach pain, tremor, Anemia and other blood disorders, yellow eyes and skin.
Glucophage (metformin)	Glucophage lowers the amount of sugar in your blood by decreasing sugar production and absorption and helping your body respond better to its own insulin, which promotes the burning of sugar. It does not, however, increase the body's production of insulin.	Abdominal discomfort, diarrhea, gas, headache, indigestion, nausea, vomiting, weakness, abdominal distention, abnormal stools, altered sense of taste, chest discomfort, chills, constipation, dizziness, flu-like symptoms, flushing, increased sweating, low blood sugar, light-headedness, muscle pain, nail disorders, pounding heartbeat, rash, shortness of breath, upper respiratory infection.

Diabetes Nostrum	Claim	Risk Factors
Glucotrol XL	Glucotrol controls diabetes by stimulating the pancreas to secrete more insulin. Occasionally, type 2 diabetics must take insulin injections on a temporary basis, especially during stressful periods or times of illness.	Constipation, diarrhea, dizziness, drowsiness, gas, headache, hives, itching, low blood sugar, nervousness, sensitivity to light, skin rash and eruptions, stomach pain, tremor, anemia and other blood disorders, yellow eyes and skin.
Glyburide (Micronase)	This medication controls diabetes by stimulating the pancreas to produce more insulin and by helping insulin to work better. Type 2 diabetics may need insulin injections, sometimes only temporarily during stressful periods such as illness, or on a long-term basis if an oral antidiabetic medication fails to control blood sugar.	Bloating, heartburn, nausea, anemia and other blood disorders, blurred vision, changes in taste, headache, hives, itching, joint pain, liver problems, muscle pain, reddening of the skin, skin eruptions, skin rash, yellowing of the skin.
Metaglip (glipizide+metformin; fixed combination tablet)	Metaglip helps remedy diabetes in two ways: by causing your body to release more insulin and by helping your body use insulin more effectively.	Abdominal pain, diarrhea, dizziness, headache, high blood pressure, hypoglycemia (low blood sugar), muscle pain, upper respiratory infection, nausea, urinary tract infection, vomiting.
Prandin (repaglinide)	Lowers blood glucose levels by stimulating the release of insulin from the pancreas.	Hypoglycemia, headache, dizziness, tiredness, nervousness or shakiness, rapid heartbeat, cold- and flu-like symptoms, diarrhea, joint ache, and back pain.
Precose (acarbose)	Precose works by slowing the body's digestion of carbohydrates so that blood sugar levels won't surge upward after a meal. Precose may be taken alone or in combination with certain other diabetes medications such as Diabinese, Micronase, Glucophage, and Insulin.	Gastrointestinal symptoms, such as diarrhea, cramping, abdominal pain, and increased gas production. Also headache and hyperglycemia.
Starlix	Starlix attacks the problem from the production angle, stimulating the pancreas to secrete more insulin. Starlix can be used alone or combined with another diabetes drug, called Glucophage, that tackles the other part of the problem, working to improve the body's response to whatever insulin it makes.	Back pain, diarrhea, dizziness, flu-like symptoms, joint infection, upper respiratory infection, accidental injury, bronchitis, coughing, low blood sugar.

Weight Charts

Table 1: Metropolitan Life Insurance Company, 1983 - Females

Height	Small Frame	Medium Frame	Large Frame
6'	138 to 151 lb	148 to 162 lb	158 to 179 lb
5'11"	135 to 148 lb	145 to 159 lb	155 to 176 lb
5'10"	132 to 145 lb	142 to 156 lb	152 to 173 lb
5'9"	129 to 142 lb	139 to 153 lb	149 to 170 lb
5'8"	126 to 139 lb	136 to 150 lb	146 to 167 lb
5'7"	123 to 136 lb	133 to 147 lb	143 to 163 lb
5'6"	120 to 133 lb	130 to 144 lb	140 to 159 lb
5'5"	117 to 130 lb	127 to 141 lb	137 to 155 lb
5'4"	114 to 127 lb	124 to 138 lb	134 to 151 lb
5'3"	111 to 124 lb	121 to 135 lb	131 to 147 lb
5'2"	108 to 121 lb	118 to 132 lb	128 to 143 lb
5'1"	106 to 118 lb	115 to 129 lb	125 to 140 lb
5'	104 to 115 lb	113 to 126 lb	122 to 137 lb
4'11"	103 to 113 lb	111 to 123 lb	120 to 134 lb
4'10"	102 to 111 lb	109 to 121 lb	118 to 131 lb

The ideal weights given in these tables are for ages 25 to 59. The weights assume you are wearing shoes with 1-inch heels and indoor clothing weighing 3 pounds.

Table 2: US National Center for Health Statistics - Females

Height	18-24 Yrs.	25-34 Yrs.	35-44 Yrs.	45-54 Yrs.	55-64 Yrs.
4'10"	114	123	133	132	135
4'11"	118	126	136	136	138
5'00"	121	130	139	139	142
5'01"	124	133	141	143	145
5'02"	128	136	144	146	148
5'03"	131	139	146	150	151
5'04"	134	142	149	153	154
5'05"	137	146	151	157	157
5'06"	141	149	154	160	161
5'07"	144	152	156	164	164
5'08"	147	155	159	168	167

Table 3: Metropolitan Life Insurance Company, 1983 - Male

Height	Small Frame	Medium Frame	Large Frame
6'4"	162 to 176 lb	171 to 187 lb	181 to 207 lb
6'3"	158 to 172 lb	167 to 182 lb	176 to 202 lb
6'2"	155 to 168 lb	164 to 178 lb	172 to 197 lb
6'1"	152 to 164 lb	160 to 174 lb	168 to 192 lb
6'	149 to 160 lb	157 to 170 lb	164 to 188 lb
5'11"	146 to 157 lb	154 to 166 lb	161 to 184 lb
5'10"	144 to 154 lb	151 to 163 lb	158 to 180 lb
5'9"	142 to 151 lb	148 to 160 lb	155 to 176 lb
5'8"	140 to 148 lb	145 to 157 lb	152 to 172 lb
5'7"	138 to 145 lb	142 to 154 lb	149 to 168 lb
5'6"	136 to 142 lb	139 to 151 lb	146 to 164 lb
5'5"	134 to 140 lb	137 to 148 lb	144 to 160 lb
5'4"	132 to 138 lb	135 to 145 lb	142 to 156 lb
5'3"	130 to 136 lb	133 to 143 lb	140 to 153 lb
5'2"	128 to 134 lb	131 to 141 lb	138 to 150 lb

The ideal weights given in these tables are for ages 25 to 59. The weights assume you are wearing shoes with 1-inch heels and indoor clothing weighing 5 pounds.

Table 4: US National Center for Health Statistics - Male

Height	18-24 Yrs.	25-34 Yrs.	35-44 Yrs.	45-54 Yrs.	55-64 Yrs.
5'02"	130	139	146	148	147
5'03"	135	145	149	154	151
5'04"	139	151	155	158	156
5'05"	143	155	159	163	160
5'06"	148	159	164	167	165
5'07"	152	164	169	171	170
5'08"	157	168	174	176	174
5'09"	162	173	178	180	178
5'10"	166	177	183	185	183
5'11"	171	182	188	190	187
6'00"	175	186	192	194	192
6'01"	180	191	197	198	197
6'02"	185	196	202	204	201

FRAME SIZE:

Your frame size or body build is determined by the thickness of the bones in your elbows, knees, ankles, and wrists. The Metropolitan Life Insurance Company offers this method of determining your body frame size: Extend your arm and bend your forearm upward at a 90 degree angle. With your fingers straight, turn the inside of your wrist toward your body. Place your thumb and index finger of the other hand on the two prominent bones of the elbow. Measure the space between the fingers against a ruler or a tape measure. Compare your measurement with the figures in the table below. Elbow measurements less than those given indicate a small frame; greater measurements indicate a large frame.

It is important to consider body composition. If you are muscular and athletic, you may weigh more than a sedentary person of the same height and frame size, yet you may be trim, while your sedentary counterpart may be overweight. If your weight comes from muscle, you may fall technically into the overweight category yet not be fat. However, in general, as you approach 20% or more above your desirable weight, your excess weight usually comes from fat. Body fat percentage can be determined by several methods, such as skinfold thickness, underwater weighing, total body water (hydrometry), and whole body potassium.

Bibliography

1. Donnelly R. Researching new treatments for obesity: from neuroscience to inflammation. Diabetes, Obesity and Metabolism 2003;5(1):1-4.
2. Release P. A History of Obesity. Vol. 2003 National Association to Advance Fat Acceptance.
3. Young JH. The Medical Messiahs. New Jersey: Princeton University Press, 1967.
4. Schwartz H. Never Satisfied: A Cultural History of Diets, Fantasies, and Fat. New York, NY: The Free Press, 1986.
5. Prescription Drugs Expenditures in 2001: Another Year of Escalating Costs. Washington, DC: The National Institute for Health Care Management Research and Educational Foundation, 2002;19.
6. The Long Struggle for the 1906 Law. FDA Consumer 1981(June).
7. Burnie D. Changes In Medicine. In: Limited TB, ed. Milestones In Medicine. NY: Reader's Digest, 2000.
8. CDC. Chronic Disease Overview: Chronic Disease Overview. Vol. 2003. Bethesda, MD, 2003.
9. Oncology DoM. Online Medical Dictionary. Vol. 2003 University of Newcastle upon Tyne, 1999.
10. Services DoD. Health Expenditures. Hyattsville, MD: National Center for Health Statistics, 2002.
11. Young JH. American Health Quackery: Collected Essays. Princeton, New Jersey: Princeton University Press, 1992.
12. Galaburda AM, Kosslyn SM, Christen Y, eds. The Languages of the Brain. Cambridge, MA: Harvard University Press, 2002.
13. Taylor RN, McEntegart DJ, Stillman EC. Statistical Techniques To Detect Fraud and Other Data Irregularities in Clinical Questionnaire Data. Drug Information Journal 2002;36(1):115-125.
14. Pearson H. Fat is spreading: Obesity epidemic sweeps into developing world. Nature News Service 2002.
15. Organization WH. Obesity and Overweight. Geneva: World Health Organization, 2003.
16. Flegal KM, Carroll MD, Ogden CL, Johnson CL. Prevalence and trends in obesity among U.S. adults: 1999-2000. JAMA 2002;288:1723-1727.
17. Flegal KM, Carroll MD, Kuczmarski RJ, Johnson CL. Overweight and obesity in the United States: prevalence and trends, 1960-1994. International Journal of Obesity 1998;22:39-47.
18. Staff. Survey finds 74% overweight in U.S. Los Angeles Times. Los Angeles, 1996;A13.
19. Roland Sturm P. Increases in Clinically Severe Obesity in the United States, 1986-2000. Archives of Internal Medicine 2003;163:2146-2148.
20. Diseases NIoDaDaK. Statistics Related to Overweight and Obesity. Vol. 2003 National Institutes of Health, 2003.
21. Nayga RM. Sociodemographic factors associated with obesity in the USA. Journal of Consumer Studies and Home Economics 1999;23(3):161-164.
22. Micic D. Obesity in children and adolescents -- a new epidemic? Journal of Pediatric Endocrinology 2001;14:1345-1352.
23. Public Health Service OotSG. The Surgeon General's Call To Action To Prevent and Decrease Overweight and Obesity 2001. Rockville, MD: U.S. Department of Health and Human Services, 2001.

24. Kiess W, Galler A, Reich A, Muller G, T.Kapellen, Deutscher J, Raile K, Kratzsch J. Clinical aspects of obesity in childhood and adolescene. Obesity Reviews 2001;2:29-36.

25. Yanovski JA. Pediatric Obesity. Reviews of Endocrine & Metabolic Disorders 2001;2001(2):371-383.

26. Dietz WH. Medical consequences of obesity in children and adolescents. In: Fairburn CG, Brownell KD, eds. Eating Disorders and Obesity: A Comprehensive Handbook. New York, NY: Guilford Press, 2002;473-476.

27. Fairburn CG, Doll HA, Welch SL, Hay PJ, Davies BA, O'Connor ME. Risk factors for binge eating disorder: A communitybased, case-controlled study. Arch General Psych 1998;55:425-432.

28. Organization WH. World Health Organization: Obesity: Preventing and Managing the Global Epidemic. 1998.

29. Guterman L. Obesity problems swells worldwide: researchers find explosive increase in body weight in developing countries. The Chronicle of Higher Education 2002;48(26):A18.

30. Brody T. Obesity. Nutritional Biochemistry. Second ed. New York, NY: Academic Press, 1999;379-420.

31. Tremblay A, Doucet E. Obesity: a disease or a biological adaptation? Obesity Reviews 2000;1(1):27-35.

32. Loos RJF, Bouchard C. Obesity - is it a genetic disorder? Journal of Internal Medicine 2003;254:401-425.

33. Filozof C, Gonzalez C. Predictors of weight gain: the biological-behavioural debate. Obesity Reviews 2000;1(1):21-26.

34. Anderson K, Kannel W. Obesity and disease. In: Bjorntorp P, Brodoff B, eds. Obesity. Philadelphia, PA: J. B. Lippincott Co, 1992;465-473.

35. Sorensen TIA. Weight loss causes increased mortality: pros. Obesity Reviews 2003;4:3-7.

36. Montague CT, O'Rahilly S. The Perils of Portliness. Diabetes 2000;49:883-888.

37. Hausman DB, DiGirolamo M, Bartness TJ, Hausman GJ, Martin RJ. The biology of white adipocyte proliferation. Obesity Reviews 2001;2:239-254.

38. Bjorntorp P. Size, number and function of adipose tissue cells in human obesity. Horm Metab Res 1974;4:77-83.

39. Hirsch J, Fried S, Edens N, RL. L. The fat cell. Med Clin N Am 1989;73:83-96.

40. Bonnet F. Fat cell size and number in obese children. In: Bonnet F, ed. Adipose Tissue in Childhood. Boca Raton, FL: CRC Press, 1981;133-154.

41. Farrakhan ML. Minister Farrakhan calls on the entire Black Nation to Declare War On Obesity (fat)! The Final Call 1996;15(20):19.

42. Mayer J. Appetite And Obesity. Food: Readings from Scientific American. San Francisco: W.H. Freeman, 1956;21-26.

43. Williams R. Obesity Is Causing Heart Problems Among the Young. The Wall Street Journal. Wednesday ed. New York, 2002;B1.

44. Dixon JB, Schachter LM, O'Brien PE. Sleep Disturbance and Obesity: Changes Following Surgically Induced Weight Loss. Arch Intern Med 2001;161(1):102-106.

45. Groop L, Orho-Melander M. The dysmetabolic syndrome. Journal of Internal Medicine 2001;250(2):105-120.

46. Case CC, Jones PH, Nelson K, O'Brian Smith E, Ballantyne CM. Impact of weight loss on the metabolic syndrome. Diabetes, Obesity and Metabolism 2002;4(6):407-414.

47. Hillis AP, Henning EM, Byrne NM, Steele JR. The biomechanics of adiposity -- structural and functional limitations of obesity and implications for movement. Obesity Reviews 2002;3:35-43.

48. Statistics BoT. National Transportation Statistics 2001. Washington, DC: U.S. Department of Transportation, 2002.

49. Kolotkin RL, Meter K, Williams GR. Quality of life and obesity. Obesity Reviews 2001;2:21--229.

50. Peltonen M, Lindroos AK, Torgerson JS. Musculoskeletal pain in the obese: a comparison with a general population and long-term changes after conventional and surgical obesity treatment. Pain 2003;104(3):549-557.

51. Martha L. Daviglus M, PhD, Kiang Liu P, Lijing L. Yan P, MPH, Amber Pirzada M, Daniel B. Garside B, Linda Schiffer M, MPH, Alan R. Dyer P, Philip Greenland M, Jeremiah Stamler M. Body Mass Index in Middle Age and Health-Related Quality of Life in Older Age. Archives of Internal Medicine 2003;163(20):2448-2455.

52. Kolotkin RL, Crosby RD, Williams GR. Health-related quality of life varies among obese subgroups. Obes Res 2002;10(8):748-756.

53. Felber JP, Golay A. Pathways from obesity to diabetes. Int J Obes Relat Metab Disord 2002;26(Suppl 2):S39-45.

54. Lewis C. Diabetes: A Growing Public Health Concern. FDA Consumer magazine. Bethesda, MD: Food and Drug Administration, 2002.

55. Astrup A, Finer N. Redefining Type 2 Diabetes: 'Diabesity' or "Obesity" Dependent Diabetes Mellitus'? Obesity Reviews 2000;1:57-59.

56. 76-1021 PN. Report of the United States National Commission on Diabetes to the Congress of the United States. Bethesda, MD: U.S. Department of Heath, Education and Welfare, 1975.

57. Kaufman FR. Type 2 Diabetes in Children and Youth. Reviews in Endocrine & Metabolic Disorders 2003;4:33-42.

58. Pinhas-Hamiel O, Dolan LM, Daniels SR, Staniford D, Khoury PR, Zeitler P. Increased incidence of non-insulin-dependent diabetes mellitus among adolescents. Journal of Pediatrics 1996;128:608-615.

59. Silverstein JH, Rosenbloom AL. Type 2 diabetes in children. Current Diabetes Report. 2001;1:19-27.

60. Statistics NCfH. National Diabetes Fact Sheet. Bethesda: CDC, 2002.

61. Anderson JW, Kendall CWC, Jenkins DJA. Importance of Weight Management in Type 2 Diabetes: Review with Meta-analysis of Clinical Studies. Journal of the American College of Nutrition 2003;22(5):331-339.

62. Case CC, Maldonado M. Diabetic ketoacidosis associated with Metabolife: a report of two cases. Diabetes, Obesity and Metabolism 2002;4(6):402-406.

63. Salmeron J, Hu FB, Manson JE, Stampfer MJ, Colditz GA, Rimm EB, Willett WC. Dietary fat intake and risk of type 2 diabetes in women. Am J Clin Nutr 2001;73(6):1019-1026.

64. Mayers D. Diabetes Diet War. U. S. News & World Report. Vol. 135, 2003;48-49.

65. Michaud DS, Liu S, Giovannucci E, Willett WC, Colditz GA, Fuchs CS. Dietary Sugar, Glycemic Load, and Pancreatic Cancer Risk in a Prospective Study. J Natl Cancer Inst 2002;94(17):1293-1300.

66. Salmeron J, Ascherio A, Rimm EB, Colditz GA, Spiegelman D, Jenkins DJ, Stampfer MJ, Wing AL, Willett WC. Dietary fiber, glycemic load, and risk of NIDDM in men. Diabetes Care 1997;20(4):545-550.

67. Murphy SP, Johnson RK. The scientific basis of recent US guidance on sugars intake. Am J Clin Nutr 2003;78:827S-833.

68. Myslobodsky M. Gourmand savants and environmental determinants of obesity. Obesity Reviews 2003;4:121-128.

69. Jenkins DJ, Kendall CW, Augustin LS, Franceschi S, Hamidi M, Marchie A, Jenkins AL, Axelsen M. Glycemic index: overview of implications in health and disease. Am J Clin Nutr 2002;76(1):266S-273.

70. Muhammad KA. Nut Poisons Described. Nuts Are Not Good for Humans. Newark, Delaware: TechDoc, Inc., 2000;31-39.

71. Jiang R, Manson JE, Stampfer MJ, Liu S, Willett WC, Hu FB. Nut and Peanut Butter Consumption and Risk of Type 2 Diabetes in Women. JAMA 2002;288(20):2554-2560.

72. Longnecker MP, Daniels JL. Environmental Contaminants as Etiologic Factors for Diabetes. Environmental Health Perspectives 2001;109(suppl 6):871-876.

73. van Dam RM, Willett WC, Rimm EB, Stampfer MJ, Hu FB. Dietary Fat and Meat Intake in Relation to Risk of Type 2 Diabetes in Men Diabetes Care 2002;25(3):417-424.

74. A.G S. Chlorinated hydrocarbon insecticides. In: Hayes WJ, Laws ER, eds. Handbook of Pesticides Toxicology. San Diego, CA: Academic Press Inc., 1991;715-915.

75. Agency UEP. Biosolids Generation, Use and Disposal in the United States. EPA530-R-99-009. Washington, DC: US Environmental Protection Agency, 1999.

76. Michalek JE, Akhtar FZ, Kiel JL. Serum Dioxin, Insulin, Fasting Glucose, and Sex Hormone-Binding Globulin in Veterans of Operation Ranch Hand. J Clin Endocrinol Metab 1999;84(5):1540-1543.

77. Remillard RbJ, Bunce NJ. Linking Dioxins to Diabetes: Epidemiology and Biological Plausibility. Environmental Health Perspectives 2002;110(9):853-858.

78. Calvert G, Sweeney M, Deddens J, Wall D. Evaluation of diabetes mellitus, serum glucose, and thyroid function among United States workers exposed to 2,3,7,8-tetrachlorodibenzo-p- dioxin. Occup Environ Med 1999;56(4):270-276.

79. Chevrier J, Dewailly E, Ayotte P, Mauriège P, Després JP, Tremblay A. Body weight loss increases plasma and adipose tissue concentrations of potentially toxic pollutants in obese individuals. Int J Obes 2000;24:1272-1278.

80. Pelletier C, Imbeault P, Tremblay A. Energy balance and pollution by organochlorines and polychlorinated biphenyls. Obesity Reviews 2003;4:17-24.

81. Muhammad E. How To Eat To Live. Vol. 1. Chicago, IL: Final Call Publishing Company, 1967.

82. Ephesians 6:11. In: C.I. Scofield DD, ed. The Holy Bible. New Scofield Reference Edition ed. New York: Oxford University Press, 1967.

83. Consultation JWFE. Diet, Nutrition and the Prevention of Chronic Diseases. WHO Technical Report Series. Geneva, Switzerland: World Health Organization, 2003.

84. Service ER. U.S. Food Expenditures by families and individuals, selected years, 1929-2001. Vol. 2003. Washington, D.C.: U.S. Department of Agriculture, 2003.

85. Blisard N, Lin B-H, Cromartie J, Ballenger N. America's Changing Appetite: Food Consumption and Spending to 2020. Food Review. Vol. 25. Washington, D.C.: Economic Research Service, USDA, 2003.

86. Gallo AE. The Food Marketing System in 1995. Agriculture Information Bulletin. Vol. 731 U.S. Department of Agriculture, Economic Research Service, Food and Consumer Economics Division., 1996.

87. Harris JM. Food Product Introductions Continue To Decline in 2000. Food Review. Vol. 25. Washington, D.C.: Economic Research Service, USDA, 2003;24-27.

88. Tillotson JE. We're Fat and Getting Fatter! What Is The Food Industry's Role. Nutrition Today 2002;37(3):136-138.

89. Gallo AE. Food and Food advertising in the United States. America's Eating Habits: Changes and Consequences. Rural Economics Division, Economic Research Service, US Department of Agriculture, 1998.

90. Schwartz MB, Puhl R. Childhood obesity: a societal problem to solve. Obesity Reviews 2003;4:57-71.

91. Horgen KB, Choate M, Brownell KD. Television food advertising: Targeting children in a toxic environment. Sage:. In: Singer DG, Singer JL, eds. Handbook of Children and the Media. Thousand Oaks, CA: Sage, 2001;447-461.

92. McNeal J. Kids as customers: a handbook of marketing to children. Lexington, MA: Lexington Books, 1992.

93. Committee DMIC. Diabetes Prevention Program Meeting Summary. National Institute of Diabetes and Digestive and Kidney Diseases, 2001.

94. Pittman QJ. Hypothalamus. Encyclopedia of Human Biology. Vol. 4 Academic Press, 1991;303-312.

95. Richards DG, McMillin DL, Mein EA, Nelson CD. Gold and Its Relationship to Neurological/Glandular Conditions. International Journal of Neuroscience 2002;112:31-53.

96. Bergen HT, Monkman N, Mobbs CV. Injection with gold thioglucose impairs sensitivity to glucose: evidence that glucose-responsive neurons are important for long-term regulation of body weight. Brain Research 1999;734:332-336.

97. Challet E, Bernard DJ, Turek FW. Gold-thioglucose-induced hypothalamic lesions inhibit metabolic modulation of light-induced circadian phase shifts in mice. Brain Research 1999;824:18-27.

98. Rolls E. Taste and olfactory processing in the brain and its relation to the control of eating. Crit Rev Neurobiol 1997;11:263-287.

99. J. Nasser P. Taste, food intake and obesity. Obesity Reviews 2001;2:213-218.

100. Ash MaI. Handbook of Food Additives: An International Guide to 7,500 Products. Brookfield, VT: Gower, 1995.

101. Kalara SP, Dube MG, Pu S, Xu B, Horvath TL, Kalra PS. Interacting Appetite-Regulating Pathways in the Hypothalamic Regulation of Body Weight. Endocrine Reviews 20(1): 68-100 1999;20(1):68-100.

102. Bradbury J. Adipocyte research may lead to new antidiabetic drugs. The Lancet 2002;359:51.

103. CFSAN. Food Additives. FDA/IFIC Brochure: U. S. Food and Drug Administration, 1992.

104. Health. Fast food 'as addictive as heroin'. BBC News. Vol. 2004, 2003.

105. Yang D, Fontaine KR, Wang C, Allison DB. Weight loss causes increased mortality: cons. Obesity Reviews 2003;4:9-16.

106. Allan Geliebter P. Strength Training Following Gastric Bypass for Obesity. New York, NY: NY Obesity Research Center, St. Luke's-Roosevelt Hospital, Columbia University, 2003.

107. Gary R Hunter P, Paul A Zuckerman M, David Bryan M. Exercise Training in Obesity-prone Black and White Women. Birmingham, Alabama: University of Alabama at Birmingham, 2003.

108. Investigating the Use of Quercetin on Glucose Absorption in Obesity, and Obesity with Type 2 Diabetes. Bethesda, MD: National Institute of Diabetes and Digestive and Kidney Diseases (NIDDK), 2003.

109. Serdula M, Mokdad A, Williamson D, Galuska D, Mendlein J, Health G. Prevalence of attempting weight loss and strategies for controlling weight. JAMA 1999;282:1353-1358.

110. Fad diets: look before you leap. Food Insight 2000;March/April:1, 4, 5.

111. Freedman M, King J, Kennedy E. Popular diets: a scientific review. Obes Res 2001;9(Supplement 1):1S - 40S.

112. National Nutrition Monitoring and Related Research Act of 1990, 1. 101st Congress. 2 ed, 1990.

113. Institute NC. Memorandum of Understanding Between Department of Health and Human Services and Department of Agriculture. Washington, D.C.: HHS, 2000.

114. Fund WCR. Food, Nutrition and the Prevention of Cancer: a Global Perspective. Washington, DC: American Institute for Cancer Research, 1997.

115. Astrup A, Grunwald G, Melanson E, Saris W, Hill J. The role of low-fat diets in body weight control: a meta-analysis of ad libitum dietary intervention studies. Int J Obes 2000;24:1545-1552.

116. Ayyad C, Andersen T. Long-term efficacy of dietary treatment of obesity: a systematic review of studies published between 1931 and 1999. Obesity Reviews 2000;1(2):113-119.

117. Editorial. What diets should we be recommending for obesity. Obes Res 2003;4:77-78.

118. Willett WC. Dietary fat plays a major role in obesity: no. Obesity Reviews 2002;3(2):59-68.

119. Sours HE, Frattali VP, Brand D, Feldman RA, Forbes AL, Swanson ALP. Sudden death associated with very low calorie weight reduction regimens. Am J Clin Nutr 1981;34:453-461.

120. Swinburn B, Egger G. Preventive strategies against weight gain and obesity. Obesity Reviews 2002;3:289-301.

121. Pharmaceutical Industry 2003. Washington, DC: Pharmaceutical Research and Manufacturers of America (PhRMA), 2003.

122. The U.S. Market for Nutraceutical Foods and Beverages. Vol. 2003 MarketResearch.com, 2002.

123. GAO. Prescription Drugs, FDA Oversight of Direct-to-Consumer Advertising Has Limitations. Washington, DC: U.S. General Accounting Office, 2002.

124. Bray GA, Greenway FL. Current and Potential Drugs for Treatment of Obesity. Endocrine Reviews 1999;20(6):805-875.

125. Putnam JJ. Cases of myxedema and acromegalia treated with benefit by sheep's thyroids: recent observations respecting the pathology of the cachexias following disease of the thyroid; clinicalrelationships of Graves's disease and acromegalia. Am J Med Sci 1893;106:125-148.

126. Masserman JH, Goldsmith H. Dinitrophenol: its therapeutic and toxic actions in certain types of psychobiologic underactivity. JAMA 1934;102:523-525.

127. Lesses MF, Myerson A. Human autonomic pharmacology. XVI. Benzedrine sulfate as an aid in the treatment of obesity. NEngl J Med 1938;218:119-124.

128. Kramer MS, Lane DA. Aminorex, dexfenfluramine, and primary pulmonary-hypertension. J Clin Epidemiol 1998;51:361-364.

129. Perchenet L, Hilfiger L, Mizrahi J, Clement-Chomienne O. Effects of Anorexinogen Agents on Cloned Voltage-Gated K+ Channel hKv1.5. J Pharmacol Exp Ther 2001;298(3):1108-1119.

130. Connolly HM, Crary JL, McGoon MD, Hensrud DD, Edwards BS, Edwards WD, Schaff HV. Valvular heart disease associated with fenfluramine-phentermine. N Engl J Med 1997;337:581-588.

131. Collins P, Williams G. Drug treatment of obesity: from past failures to future successes? British Journal of Clinical Pharmacology 2001;51(1):13-25.

132. Kinnell HG. European withdrawal of appetite suppressants. Obesity Reviews 2003;4:79-81.

133. Batterham RL, Cohen MA, Ellis SM, Le Roux CW, Withers DJ, Frost GS, Ghatei MA, Bloom SR. Inhibition of Food Intake in Obese Subjects by Peptide YY3-36. N Engl J Med 2003;349(10):941-948.

134. Stinson SC. Fine Chemical: Last year saw disappointing growth in both pharmaceutical and agricultural fine chemicals; firms and academics continue to create new technology. Chemical & Engineering News 2001;79(28):65-84.

135. Report I. Danger At The Drugstore. U.S. News & World Report, 1996;47-53.

136. Report I. Drug Alert! U.S. News & World Report, 1995;49-54.

137. Hunter BT. Some Foods and Drugs Don't Mix. Consumer Research 1996;79(8):19-21.
138. Dahan A, Altman H. Food - drug interaction: grapefruit juice augments drug bioavailability - mechanism, extent and relevance. European Journal of Clinical Nutrition 2004;58:1-9.
139. Rouhi AM. CUSTOM CHEMICALS: Custom producers of pharmaceutical active ingredients and advanced intermediates continue to adjust to challenging economic conditions. Chemical & Engineering News 2003;81(7):55-73.
140. Narbro K, Agren G, Jonsson E, Naslund I, Sjostrom L, Peltonen M. Pharmaceutical Costs in Obese Individuals: Comparison With a Randomly Selected Population Sample and Long-term Changes After Conventional and Surgical Treatment: The SOS Intervention Study. Arch Intern Med 2002;162(18):2061-2069.
141. Fee E. The origins and development of public health in the United States. In: Detels R, Holland WW, McEwen J, Omenn GS, eds. Oxford Textbook of Public Health. New York: Oxford University Press, 1997.
142. Blair DF, Haines LW. Mortality experience according to build at higher durations. Society of Actuaries 1966;18:35-46.
143. Conference PoaNIoHCD. Gastrointestinal surgery for severe obesity. Am J Clin Nutr 1992;55(Supplement 2):487S-619S.
144. Rationale for the Surgical Treatment of Morbid Obesity. American Society for Bariatric Surgery, 2001.
145. Genton L, Kudsk KA. Interactions between the enteric nervous system and the immune system: role of neuropeptides and nutrition. The American Journal of Surgery 2003;186(3):253-258.
146. Michael D. Gershon MD. The Second Brain. New York, NY: Harper Collins Publishers, 1998.
147. Piotrowski J. Obesity surgery brings profits; Forest Health opens sixth acute-care facility. Modern Healthcare 2002.
148. Diseases. NIoDaDaK. Gastric Surgery for Severe Obesity. NIH Publication No. 96-4006, April 1996.
149. Editorial. Laparoscopic gastric bypass an option for the obese. AORN Journal 2002;75(2):346.
150. National Heart L, and Blood Institute. Clinical Guidelines on the Identification, Evaluation, and Treatment of Obesity in Adults: The Evidence Report. NHLBI Obesity Education Initiative Expert Panel on the Identification, Evaluation, and Treatment of Obesity in Adults. Washington, DC: U.S. Department of Health and Human Services, 1998.
151. Association AO. Shape Up America! Guidance for the Treatment of Adult Obesity. Bethesda, MD: American Obesity Association, 1998.
152. IBSR. IBSR 2000-2001 Winter Pooled Report. Iowa City: International Bariatric Surgery Registry, 2001;19.
153. Sundbom M, Hedenstrom H, Gustavsson S. Duodenogastric bile reflux after gastric bypass: a cholescintigraphic study. Dig Dis Sci. 2002;47(8):1891-6.
154. Williamson JS, Wyandt CM. Herbal therapies: The facts and the fiction. Drug Topics 1997(August 04).
155. Garrard J, Harms S, Eberly LE, Matiak A. Variations in Product Choices of Frequently Purchased Herbs: Caveat Emptor. Arch Intern Med 2003;163(19):2290-2295.
156. Draves AH, Walker SE. Analysis of the hypericin and pseudohypericin content of commercially available St John's Wort preparations. The Canadian Journal of Clinical Pharmacology 2003;10, Number 3: 114-11(3):114-118.
157. Muller MJ, Mast M, Asbeck I, Langnase K, Grund A. Prevention of obesity - is it possible? Obesity Reviews 2001;2(1):15-28.

158. Dhabi A, Daniel KS. Middle East leads the world in obesity. Gulf News Online Edition. DUBAI, United Arab Emirates, 2001.

159. Wright K. Staying Alive. Discover. Vol. 24, 2003;64-70.

160. Weindruch RH, ed. Effects of Dietary Restriction on Aging. Frontiers in Longevity Research. Springfield, IL: Charles C. Thomas Publishers, 1992.

161. Barnett M, Collier GR, Zimmet P, O'Dea K. The Effect of Restricting Energy Intake on Diabetes in Psammomys Obesus. International Journal of Obesity 1994;18:789-794.

162. Dunne LJ, ed. Nutrition Almanac. 3 ed. New York: McGraw-Hill, 1990.

163. Overweight? -- New Facts You Need To Know. U.S. News and World Report, 1959;68-70.

164. Fritsch J. Scientists Unmask Diet Myth: Willpower. The New York Times. Late ed, 1999;1.

165. just-food.com. Lack of time to blame for poor eating habits in children - research. Vol. 2003. UK: Aroq Ltd, 2003.

166. Prentice AM, Jebb SA. Fast foods, energy density and obesity: a possible mechanistic link. Obesity Reviews 2003;4(4):187-194.

167. Vermunt SHF, Pasman WJ, Schaafsma G, Kardinaal AFM. Effects of sugar intake on body weight: a review. Obesity Reviews 2003;4:91-99.

168. Smith AG, Gangolli SD. Organochlorine chemicals in seafood: occurrence and health concerns. Food and Chemical Toxicology 2002;40(6):767-779.

169. Muhammad KA. Large Fish? FAQs About How To Eat To Live. Vol. 2. Newark, DE: TechDoc, Inc., 2003;39.

170. Hunter BT. How We Spend Our Food Dollars. Consumers' Research 1995;79(2):14-15.

171. Muhammad E. Lengthen Your Life. How To Eat To Live. Vol. 2. Chicago: Muhammad's Temple of Islam No. 2, 1972;14.

172. 2002 World pharma sales growth: slower, but still healthy. IMS World Review 2003 2003.

173. Muldoon MF, Manuck SB, Matthews KA. Lowering cholesterol concentrations and mortality. BMJ 1990;301:309-314.

174. Fabricatore AN, Walden TA. Treatment of Obesity: An Overview. Clinical Diabetes 2003;21(2):67-72.

175. Perez-Martin A, Raynaud E, Mercier J. Insulin resistance and associated metabolic abnormalities in muscle: effects of exercise. Obesity Reviews 2001;2(1):47-59.

176. Dallman MF, Pecoraro N, Akana SF, Fleur SEl, Gomez F, Houshyar H, Bell ME, Bhatnagar S, Laugero KD, Manalo S. Chronic stress and obesity: A new view of "comfort food". Proceedings of the National Academy of Sciences 2003;100(20):11696-11701.

177. Jaana L, Ellen E, Ulla S. Stress-related eating and drinking behavior and body mass index and predictors of this behavior. Preventive Medicine 2002;34(1):39-39.

178. Weathers D. Why Diets Alone Don't Work. Essence. Vol. 34, 2003;188-194.

179. Björntorp P. Do stress reactions cause abdominal obesity and comorbidities? Obesity Reviews 2001;2:73-86.

180. John 2:15. In: C.I. Scofield DD, ed. The Holy Bible. New Scofield Reference Edition ed. New York: Oxford University Press, 1967.

181. Alfred JB. Will 'fat-free' lose its charm? Milling & Baking News. Vol. 74, 1996;26-28.

Index